Palliative Care

Edited by Mukadder Mollaoğlu

Published in London, United Kingdom

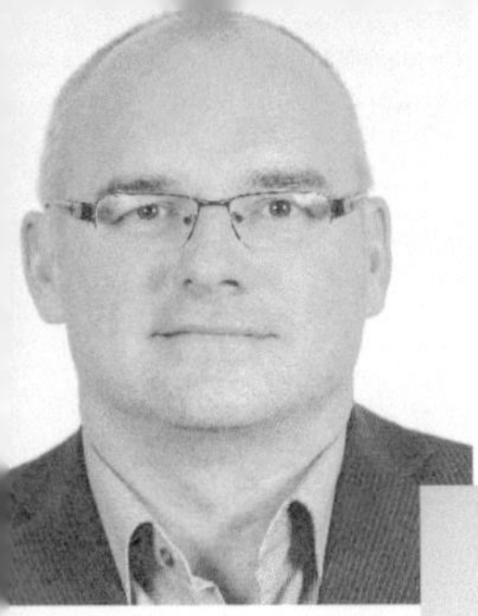
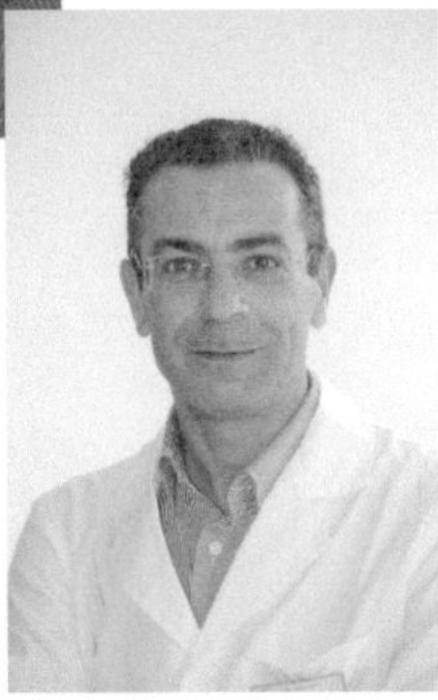
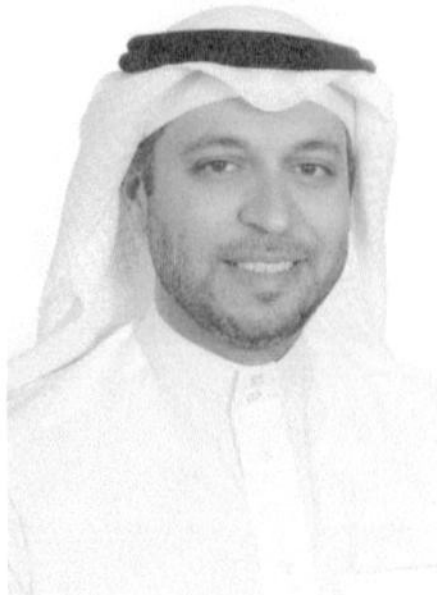
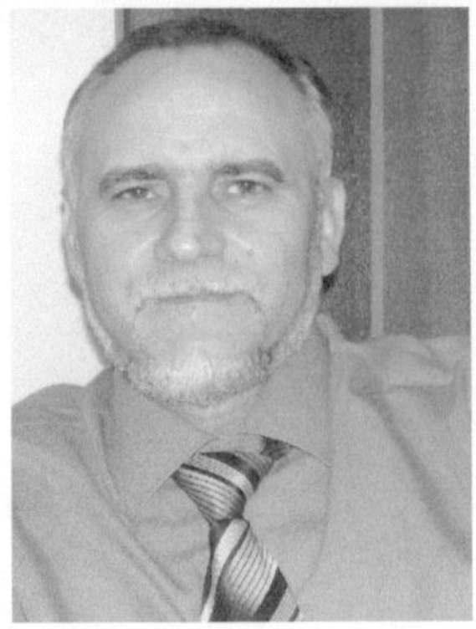
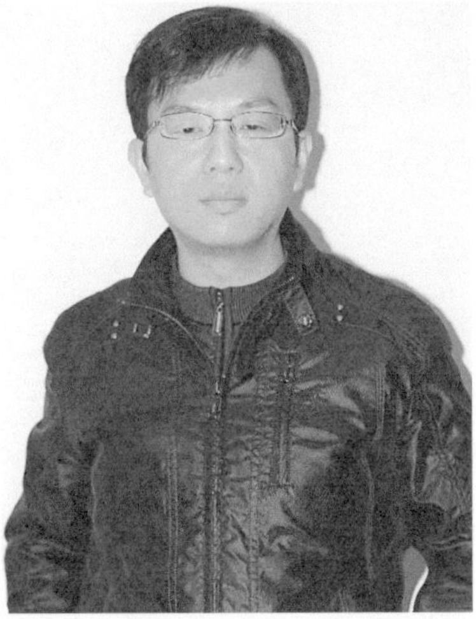
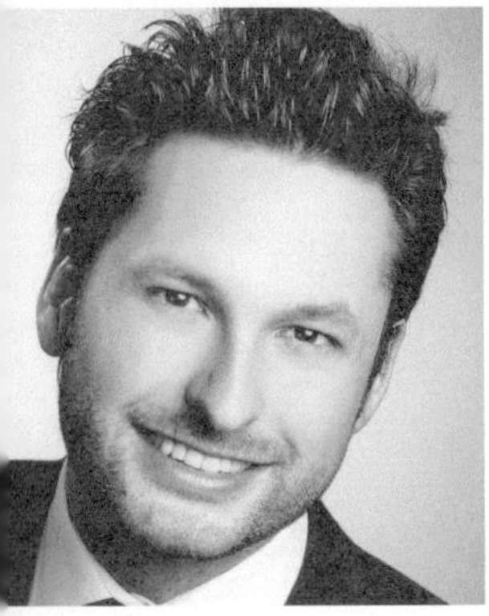
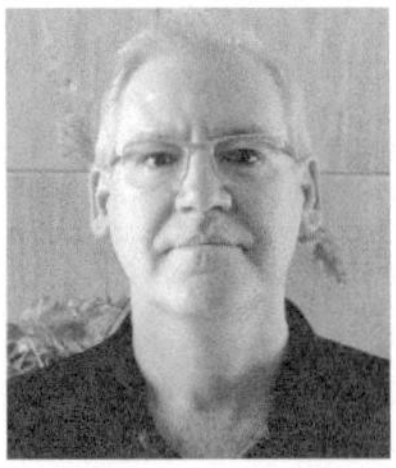

IntechOpen

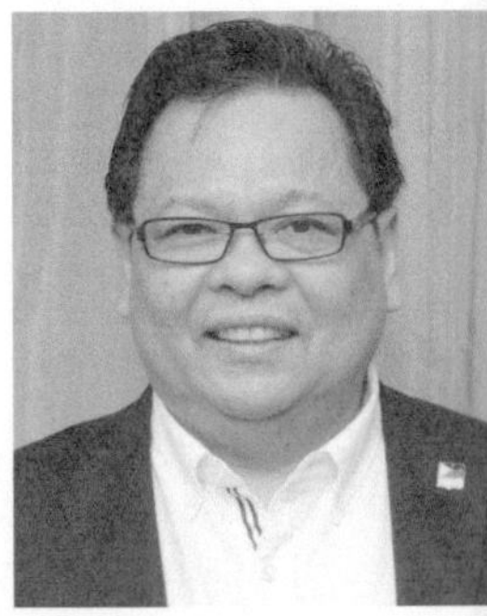
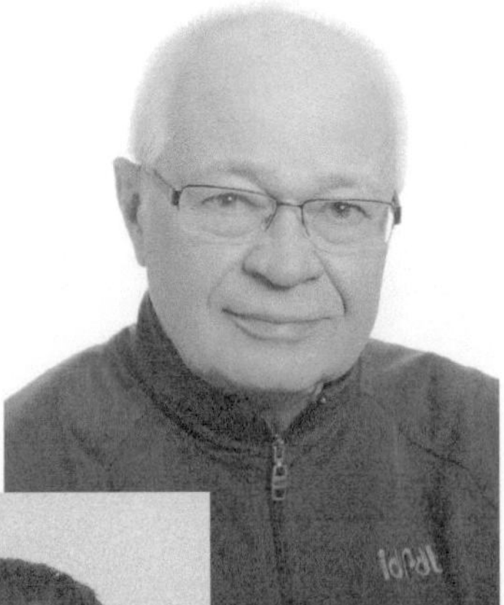
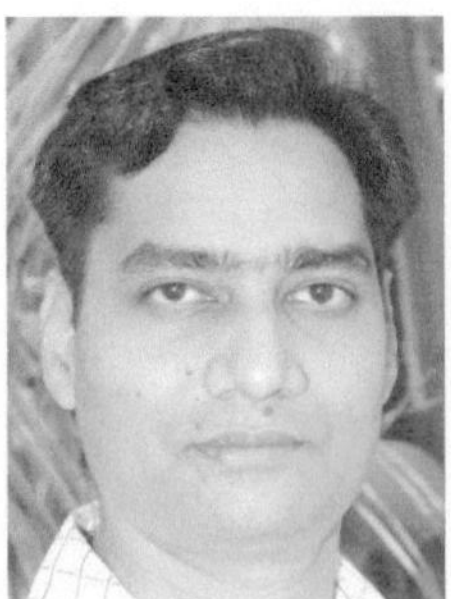
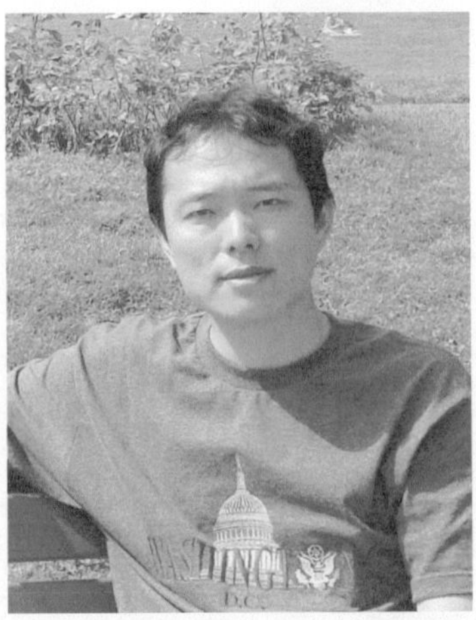
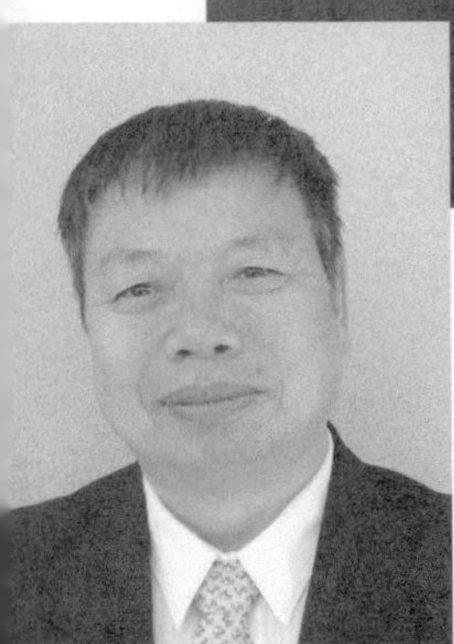
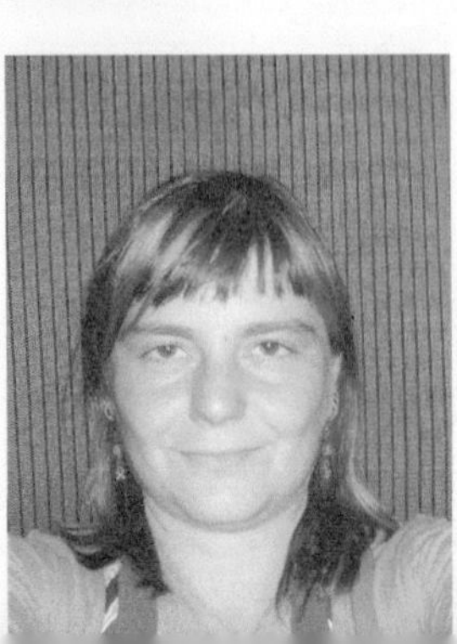

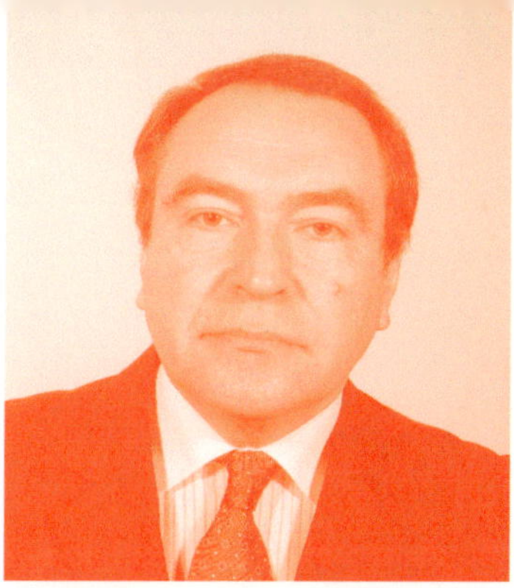

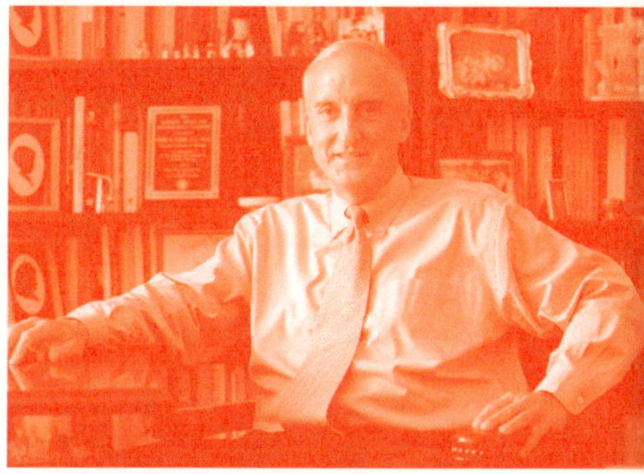

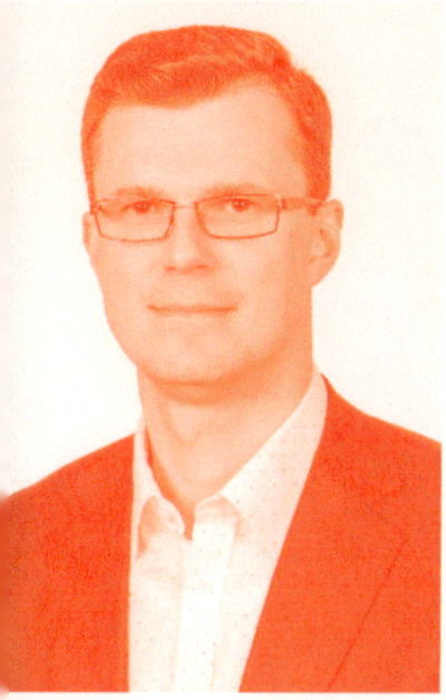

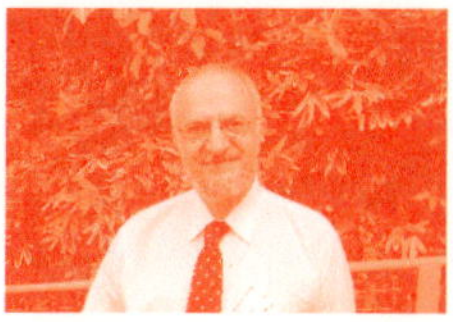

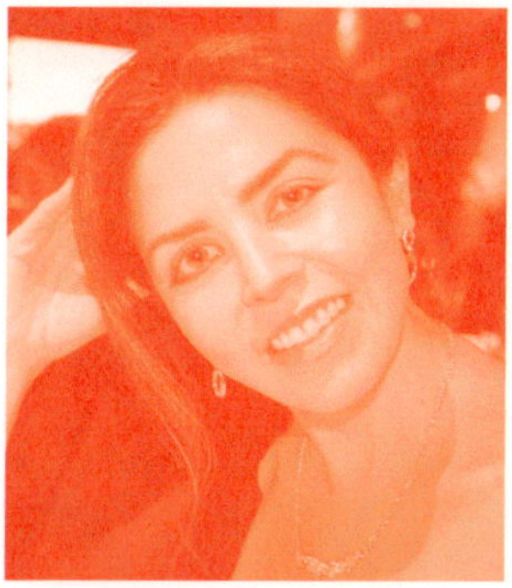

Supporting open minds since 2005

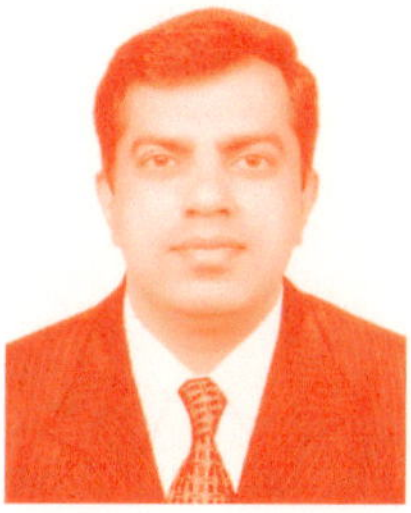

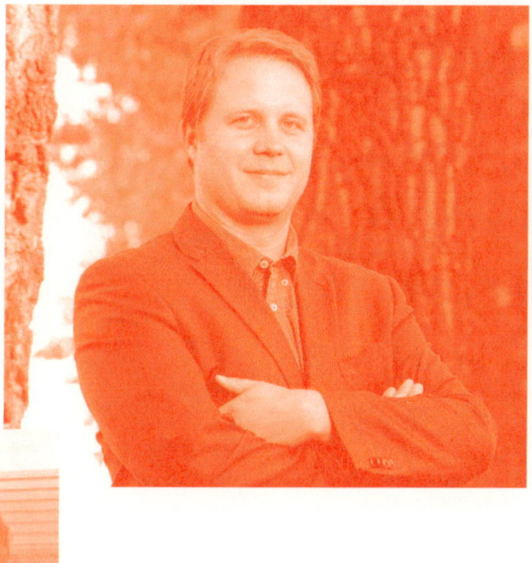

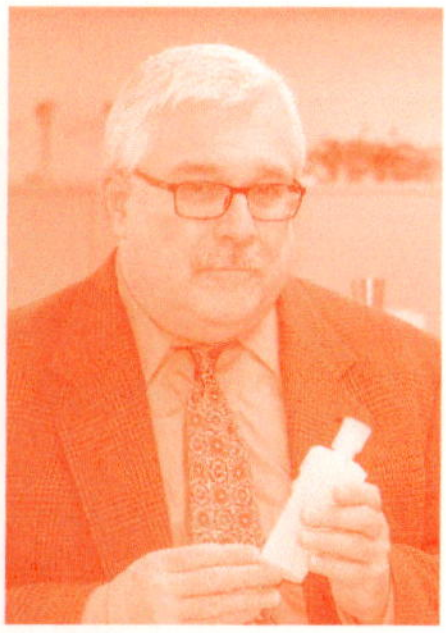

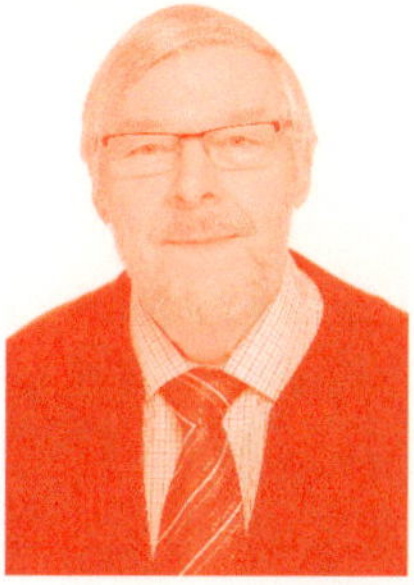

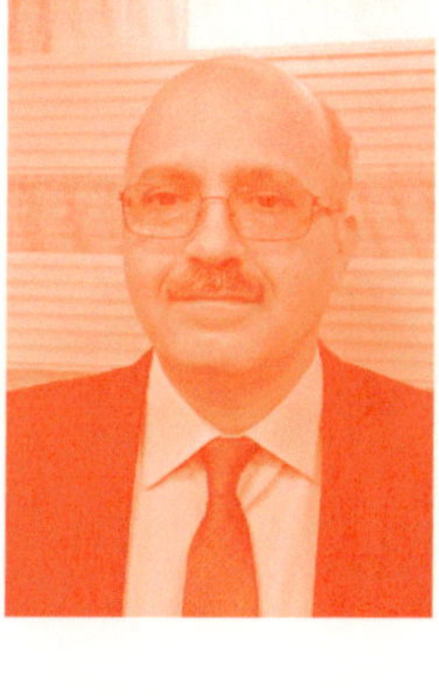

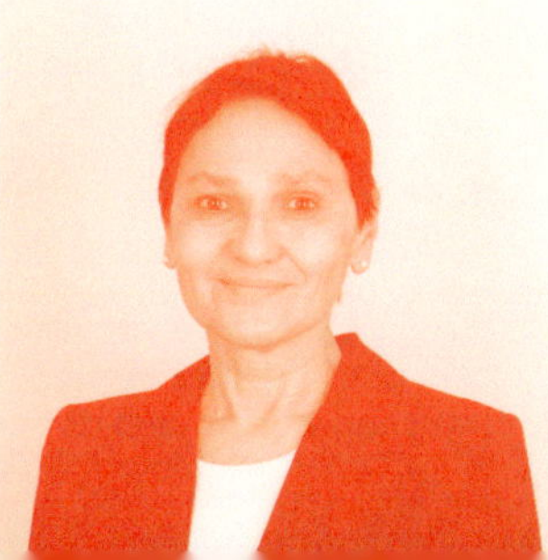

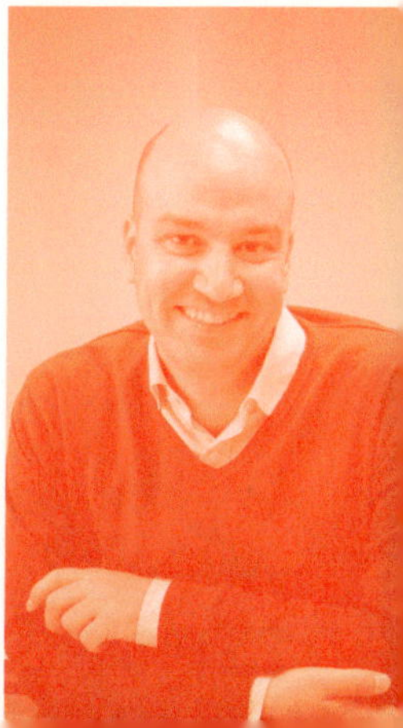

Palliative Care
http://dx.doi.org/10.5772/intechopen.77739
Edited by Mukadder Mollaoğlu

Contributors
Thomas Thaniyath, Juliana Dias Reis Pessalacia, Ana Paula Da Silva, Adriano Menis Ferreira, Jacqueline Resende Boaventura, Aires Garcia Dos Santos Júnior, Luciana Ferreira Da Silva, Juliana Guimarães Lima Munis, Habtamu Abera Areri, Richard Love, Sheikh Iqbal Ahamed, Trisha Dunning, Peter Martin, Sukru Keles, Daniel Nnadi, Swati Singh, Emmanuel Nwobodo, Yu Uneno, Soichiro Okamoto, Masanori Mori, Nobuhisa Nakajima, Takashi Yamaguchi, Georg Bollig, Mukadder Mollaoglu, Murat Can Mollaoğlu, Döne Günay

First published in London, United Kingdom, 2019 by IntechOpen
IntechOpen is the global imprint of INTECHOPEN LIMITED, registered in England and Wales, registration number: 11086078, The Shard, 25th floor, 32 London Bridge Street
London, SE19SG - United Kingdom
Printed in Croatia

British Library Cataloguing-in-Publication Data
A catalogue record for this book is available from the British Library

Additional hard and PDF copies can be obtained from orders@intechopen.com

Palliative Care
Edited by Mukadder Mollaoğlu
p. cm.
Print ISBN 978-1-78984-075-9
Online ISBN 978-1-78984-076-6
eBook (PDF) ISBN 978-1-83962-195-6

For EU product safety concerns:
IN TECH d.o.o., Prolaz Marije Krucifikse Kozulić 3, 51000 Rijeka, Croatia, info@intechopen.com or visit our website at intechopen.com.

Meet the editor

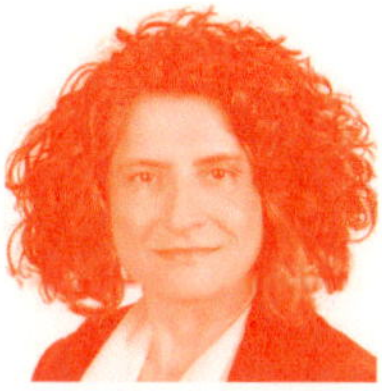

Professor Mukadder Mollaoğlu graduated from the Faculty of Health Sciences at Sivas Cumhuriyet University, Turkey, where she currently works, in 1991. She obtained a doctorate at Istanbul University Health Sciences Institute. Her research focuses on examining the effects of chronic diseases on the quality of life of patients; she also lectures and publishes in her field. She is an editorial board member and reviewer for many medical journals and has published papers in eminent journals as well as books in the field of chronic diseases and palliative care. Dr. Mollaoğlu has participated in a number of national and international panels, conferences and congresses related to quality of life, where she has held various duties such as speaker and session chairperson. She is a member of many associations on chronic diseases.

Contents

Preface

Today the number of individuals with chronic and life-threatening or incurable diseases is rapidly increasing. This has led to an increased interest among health professionals in the care of these patients and efforts to develop approaches to improve their quality of life. All these efforts have caused palliative care to become an important field of medicine despite being a relatively new discipline.

Palliative care is an organized and highly structured care philosophy and is very important in the management of many chronic diseases, especially cancer. It aims to improve the quality of life of patients with life-threatening health problems. In palliative care, pharmacological and non-pharmacological methods are used together with supportive approaches to prevent or relieve symptoms and provide a comfortable life for the patient.

The most effective way to control the occurrence of symptoms is to provide palliative care with an interdisciplinary approach. As a multidisciplinary health service, palliative care is a team effort. The palliative care team supports the patient and the patient's family to help maintain a quality life in the patient, effectively control symptoms, facilitate communication while respecting patient decisions and choices, and provide family support during the grieving process.

Palliative care is a humanitarian service that is unique to the cultural and social structure of each individual. This book describes what palliative care is, who can be given this service, where it is provided, its purpose and the policies and practices of palliative care according to different countries. This book is a significant contribution to the literature and it is my hope that it will improve the quality of life of patients with palliative care needs as well as that of their families.

PhD Mukadder Mollaoğlu
Professor,
Health Science Faculty,
Sivas Cumhuriyet University,
Sivas, Turkey

Section 1

Conceptual Aspects of Palliative Care and Different Region Applications

Chapter 1

Palliative Care Education for Everybody

Georg Bollig

Abstract

This chapter is about palliative care education for everybody including both professional health care workers and all citizens. A six-step approach to life-long palliative care education (as first described by Bollig in 2008 and published as a conference poster in 2009 and a book in German in 2010) will be proposed and discussed. The chapter will summarize the public knowledge approach to palliative care implementation (Bollig 2008) and other strategies to educate the public about palliative care. The concept of Last Aid courses for citizens will be introduced, and international experiences with this concept will be discussed. A possible combination of Last Aid courses and the compassionate community approach might improve palliative care provision in the community.

Keywords: Palliative care, worldwide, education, citizens, public health, compassionate communities, Last Aid course

1. Introduction and background

Our world is in constant change, and today, there is an enormous pressure by the mass media and the Internet to handle a massive amount of information every single day. To keep up with the current knowledge is therefore not an easy task. There is an increasing focus on life-long learning. This applies also to the field of palliative care and end-of-life care. Taking into account the increasing number of frail elderly people and people with demanding care needs in the future, it is obvious that all health care professionals should know how to provide palliative care and end-of-life care. But why should everybody be interested in learning palliative care when there are specialists to handle that? Due to an increased overall life expectancy, the demographic change and a growing awareness of palliative care needs of patients with nonmalignant diseases as, for example, terminal stages of heart-diseases, kidney diseases, neurological diseases, etc., an expected enormous number of people with a need for palliative care cannot be treated by specialized palliative care providers alone. In order to provide good palliative care to all in need, all citizens have to join in to help to provide palliative care for everybody in need. According to Kellehear, everybody has a responsibility of providing end-of-life care for others [1, 2].

Although many people would prefer to die at home, death has moved to happen mostly in institutions like hospitals or nursing homes within the last decades. Thus, communities and health care services have to prepare for an increasing number of people in need of palliative care and end-of-life care at home and in nursing homes [3–5]. The health care systems around the world will not be able to cope with this enormous task without an increased contribution from the public. In order to meet the needs of as many dying people as possible, the health care system has to cooperate with relatives, friends, and the whole community [1–4]. Based on these facts and thoughts, there is a need that everybody should be educated in palliative care in order to be capable of caring for seriously ill and dying people at home.

2. Learning palliative care throughout life for everybody

As pointed out above, the enormous need for palliative care in the future indicates a need not only to educate health care professionals about palliative care but also to include the whole society and all citizens. First Aid and emergency care can be used as an example for cooperation of the health care system and citizens. Without the help of citizens who provide first aid, many people would die or suffer from more serious damages following a heart attack, cardiac arrest, or trauma. The example of the city of Seattle in the USA has shown that the public can be trained and motivated to participate as bystanders in emergency care [6, 7]. In Seattle, 850,000 people have been trained in cardiopulmonary resuscitation (CPR) since 1971 [6]. The crucial factors to achieve that have been public education classes where people have to attend only once for a short period of approx 1–2 hours and broad information and motivation of the public [6, 7].

2.1 The public knowledge approach

Several models of implementing palliative care have been described in the literature [8, 9]. The most common used approach uses an expert to ensure a good quality of palliative care provision [8, 9]. Based on my experience from working at Harborview Medical Center in Seattle and observations from the work of Medic I and Medic II, I have adapted the approach from emergency medicine applied in Seattle to the field of palliative care. The so-called *public knowledge approach* [7, 10–13] aims to incorporate knowledge about palliative care and end-of-life care in public knowledge that everyone should have. This should in the future become an essential part of public education in schools alongside with biology and first aid education. Palliative care knowledge for the public in palliative care can in analogy with first aid be called *Last Aid*. This expression makes it clear for most people that it includes care at the end-of-life. Many people associate care at the end-of-life and a supplement to first aid with the term *Last Aid* [14]. The public knowledge approach assists implementation of palliative care in the public and may enhance knowledge about palliative care for all health care professionals and the public. It uses lay people to make palliative care available everywhere for all people in need. The *Last Aid course* forms the educational foundation of this approach in order to enable everyone to provide palliative care in the community. It may also form an essential component of the compassionate community approach [15]. The *Last Aid course* will be described in more detail under 3.

2.2 The chain of palliative care

In analogy to the chain of survival used in emergency medicine (**Figure 1**), a *chain of palliative care* (**Figure 2**) was introduced to illustrate palliative care provision in the community. The first step is that the patient himself or others (e.g. relatives, friends, and neighbors) recognize a need for palliative care. The approach is patient-centered. As in emergency care, one contact (the emergency call) should be enough to get the level of care which corresponds to the patients' needs. If a

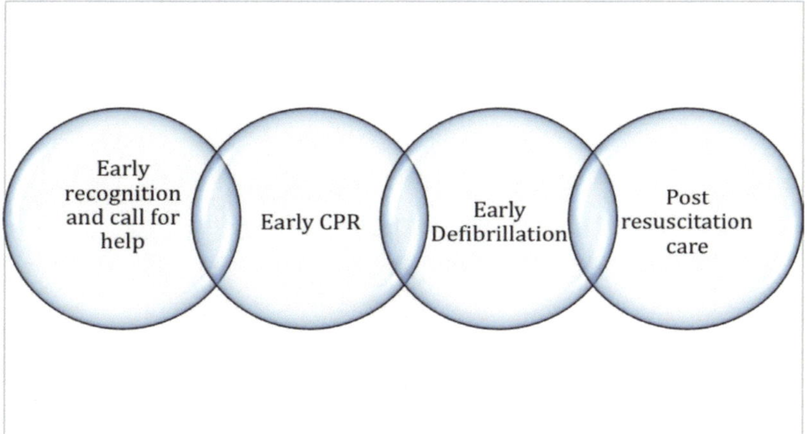

Figure 1.
The chain of survival (from emergency care).

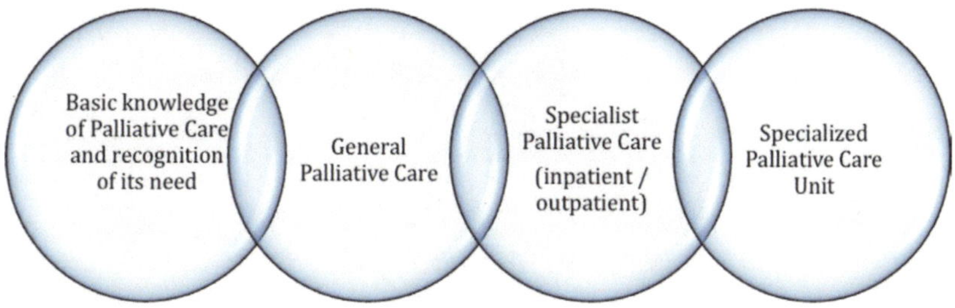

Figure 2.
The chain of palliative care.

general practitioner or a community nurse need help to treat a patient, a palliative care specialist or a specialized palliative care team should be contacted. The patient might be admitted to a specialized palliative care ward if it is not possible to provide satisfactory care within the home.

2.3 The six-step approach to education in palliative care for all

This approach (**Figure 3**) includes education for the public as initial step. One important feature is the demand for multidisciplinary education for all professionals involved in palliative care. Multidisciplinary education can be used to include a team-based approach not only in palliative care provision but also already in learning palliative care. This may increase the understanding of the different views of the different stakeholders involved in palliative care provision. Unfortunately, most education programs in palliative care for health care professionals are monodisciplinary [7]. The European Association for Palliative Care has described three levels of palliative care knowledge (A, B, and C), and educational programs have been designed for professionals (nurses, physicians, etc.) in the field of palliative care according to [16]. In order to include the public, as well as leaders and researches, the six-step approach has been modified to include six different levels. These are six steps on the ladder to education and acquisition of competence in palliative care. It is important to aim for a multidisciplinary education in order to bring the members of the future multidisciplinary teams together already during the learning phase. This will help to understand the different tasks and views of the different professions and can help a team-based approach.

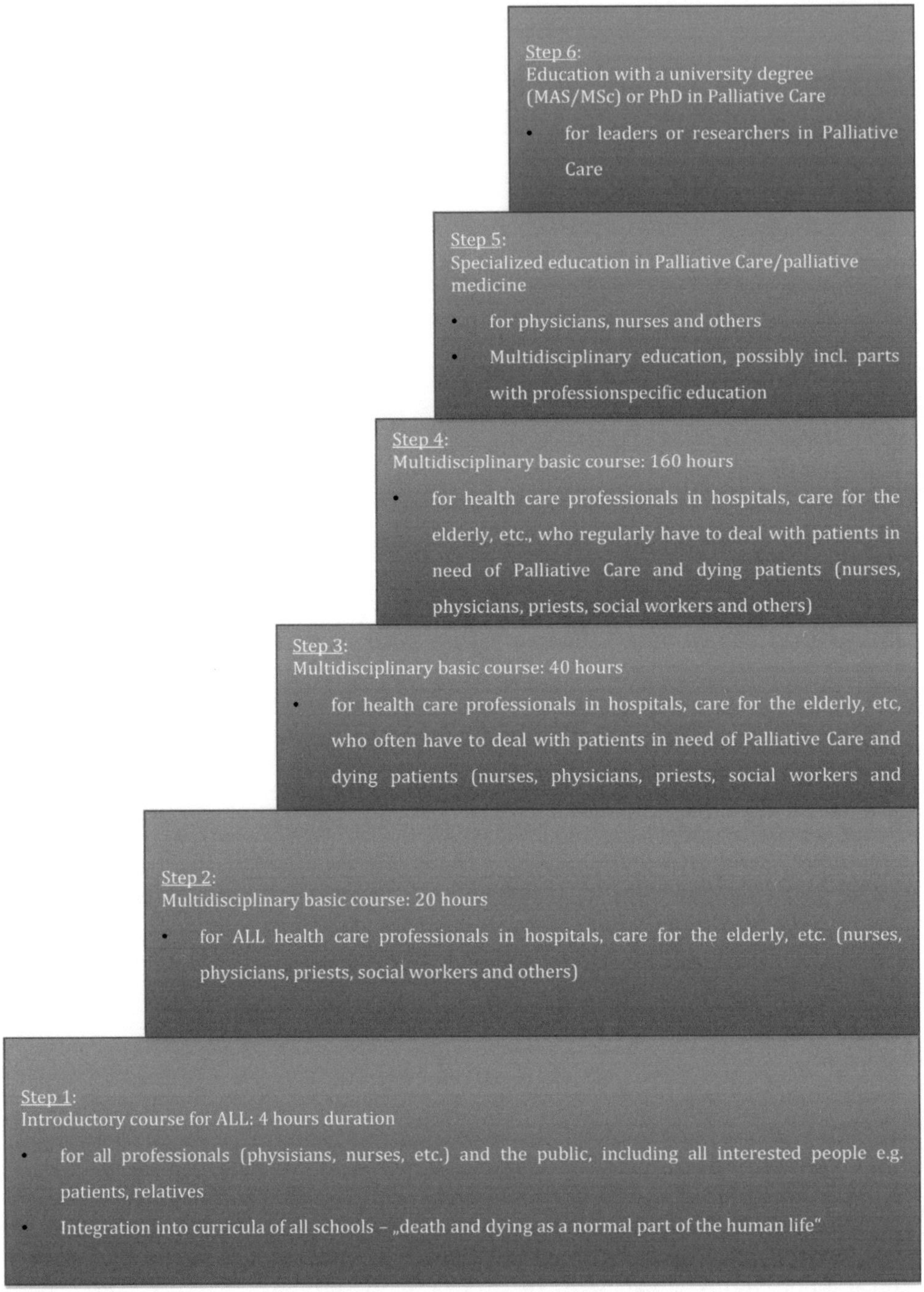

Figure 3.
The six-step approach to education in palliative care for all.

The six steps will now be explained in more detail:

- *Step 1:* Public knowledge about palliative care and end-of-life care for all citizens. Learning palliative care should start already in school. Step 1 is at the same time the basic knowledge for all health care professionals and the whole staff working in hospitals, nursing homes, and other facilities that provide medical care and sometimes palliative care. This includes also staff members working in cleaning, household, mechanics and administration, etc.

- *Step 2:* Palliative care knowledge for all health care professionals including those who do not regularly provide care for seriously ill and dying people. This is meant to ensure an adequate level of care throughout the health care service.

- *Step 3:* Health care professionals who often have to provide care for seriously ill and dying people need a good knowledge about palliative care and symptom treatment.

- *Step 4:* 160 hours of training have been suggested as appropriate for health care professionals who have to care for seriously ill and dying people on a regular basis.

- *Step 5:* A specialized education is needed for health care professionals and others whose main task is care and treatment of seriously ill and dying people. Some countries have for example already introduced a specialization or sub-specialization for physicians and nurses. This helps to ensure a high level of specialized palliative care. Also for these people, education should be as multidisciplinary as possible.

- *Step 6:* Further academic education leading to a Master or PhD degree is important for future leaders and researchers in the field of palliative care. The academic education should aim to support multidisciplinary work in teams, leadership, and research to implement new knowledge and to establish new knowledge in practice.

In Germany, the *Last Aid course* is recognized by the German Association for Palliative Medicine (DGP) and the German Hospice Association (DHPV) as first step of the education in palliative care for both lay people and professionals (personal communication). All health care professionals should have a basic education in palliative care (step 2). According to the grade of daily involvement and professional role in palliative care, the steps 3 to 6 show the educational level suggested for health care workers, leaders, and researchers in the field (**Figure 3**). The Last Aid course is designed as a joint foundation for both lay people and professionals. As for first aid courses, it is recommended to repeat the Last Aid course after a few years to keep updated with the current knowledge and practice. The international *Last Aid* working group revises the curriculum and the course presentation at present every 1 to 2 years.

3. Teaching the public

Different authors have suggested that there is a need to teach the public about palliative care [7, 10–13, 17–19]. Nevertheless, there are just a few existing projects that try to teach the public on a large scale. Approaches that have been used are for example: group teaching of family carers in Australia [20, 21] or the open formats of the so-called death café or death chat [22, 23]. The latter invite people to discuss death and dying on a drop-in basis without any obligation to participate again.

3.1 The *Last Aid course*

A model to teach the public about palliative care is the *Last Aid course*. The *Last Aid course* is a clearly structured approach (like a first aid course) where knowledge is provided, but in addition, a discussion about death and dying and a reflection of one's attitude is encouraged. An international Last Aid working group with participants from different European countries works during regular meetings every 1–2 years on a consensus about the course curriculum and content. This ensures that the *Last Aid courses* in different areas and countries are based on the same curriculum based on actual scientific knowledge and practice of palliative care. The consensus of experts from different countries ensures evidence-based and updated knowledge to be delivered to the public. An important task of the working group is to ensure that the educational format uses an everyday language in order to address the whole public. **Table 1** shows my first ideas about the topics to teach as first presented in 2008 [7].

Usually the *Last Aid course* includes four modules (each lasting 45 minutes) only. Topics included in the four modules are care at the end of life, Advance Care planning and decision making, symptom management, and cultural aspects of death and bereavement. The course is given during one afternoon or evening with four teaching units (45 minutes each). It usually consists of two parts with 1.5 hours and a 30-minute break. At present, nine European countries participate in the International *Last Aid* working group. These countries include Germany, Denmark, Austria, Switzerland, Slovenia, Scotland, Lithuania, Estonia, Bulgaria and Latvia. At present, talks with more countries about participation in the international Last Aid working group are ongoing. Some countries have already functioning systems

• Dying as a normal part of human life
• Problems around dying, e.g., troublesome symptoms, total pain concept, medical and ethical end of life decisions
• Treatment of troublesome symptoms
• Medical and nonmedical treatment options, fluid and nutrition at the end of life
• Bereavement and grief

Table 1.
Topics Last Aid course.

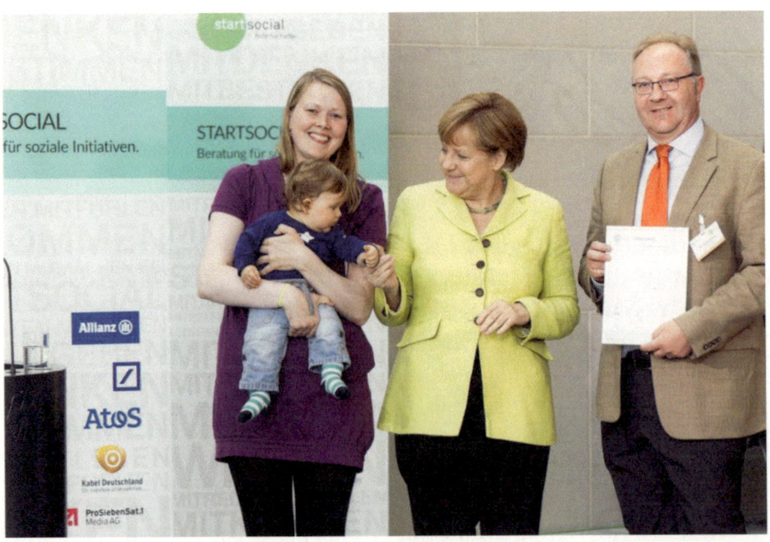

Figure 4.
Invitation to chancellor Angela Merkel 2015. (Photo: startsocial/Thomas Effinger).

for teaching *Last Aid courses* on a regular basis, while others are still in the starting phase of implementing *Last Aid* education for the public.

The first results from a German pilot-study [10] from 2015 were very positive which lead to several awards including an invitation to the chancellor Angela Merkel (**Figure 4**) [24, 25]. The scientific evaluation of the *Last Aid course* is at present ongoing in different countries and includes both teaching of the public and the use of *Last Aid courses* to teach nonmedical staff in hospitals [26]. In Germany, work with courses for children starting at the age of 8 years is in the testing phase. First results will be published on the congress of the European Association for Palliative Care [27]. In 2019, the European Association for Palliative Care has established a taskforce on Last Aid [28]. **Table 2** shows the timeline of the development of the Last Aid course project and the International Last Aid working group.

2008	First presentation of the Last Aid concept in the Master Thesis of Georg Bollig
2009	Posterpresentation 11th Congress of the European Association for Palliative Care, Vienna
2010	Master thesis published as a book
2009–2011	Development of a Last Aid Course with 16 teaching hours in cooperation with the Austrian Red Cross and the IFF Vienna, University Klagenfurt/Graz
2012	Honorable mention for the lecture "The public knowledge approach as educational concept for bringing Palliative Care to the public" International Palliative Care Network conference
2013–2014	Development of a Last Aid Course with 4 teaching hours in cooperation of the Norwegian and Danish Associations for Palliative Care with Letzte Hilfe Deutschland
2014–2015	First pilot courses in Norway, Germany and Denmark
2015	Participation in the project startsocial–Invitation to chancellor Angela Merkel
2015	Honorable mention for the posterpresentation "Teaching Palliative Care to the Public: The Last Aid Course—An International Multicentre project from Norway, Denmark and Germany" International Palliative Care Network conference
2015	Reception of an award for Palliative Care from the German Association for Palliative Medicine and the pharmaceutical company Grünenthal
2016	Symposium of the Paula-Kubitschek-Vogel Stiftung München on Last Aid
2016	Publication of a German handbook for Last Aid Course participants
2016	Lecture on Last Aid on the International Palliative Care congress in Montreal, Canada
2017	1. German Symposium on Last Aid in Hamburg
2017	Lecture on Last Aid on the Scottish Palliative Care congress in Edinburgh, Scotland
2017–2019	Last Aid International as EUPCA project
2018	Last Aid courses recognized and recommended by German Hospice Association (Deutscher Hospiz und Palliativvverband-DHPV) and the German Association for Palliative Medicine (Deutsche Gesellschaft für Palliativmedizin-DGP)
2018	Meeting of the International *Last Aid* working group in May in Frankfurt
2018	Relaunch of the German and English homepage www.lastaid.info
2018	Lecture on Last Aid on the 1. Baltic Palliative Care Conference in Liepaja, Latvia
2018	2. German Symposium on Last Aid in Kassel
2018	Publication of a Danish handbook for Last Aid Course participants

Table 2.
Timetable of the milestones and awards of the Last Aid Course project.

4. Turning knowledge into practice

Knowledge alone is not sufficient enough to change practice. This important statement from Ferris [29] should inform all efforts to spread palliative care in the community. In order to turn knowledge into practice, we do need education, reflection of own attitudes toward death and dying, and a public discussion on the topic. Without a palliative care attitude of the public informed by hospice philosophy and humanitarian thinking, it may not be possible to provide palliative care to all people who need it. From my point of view, it is therefore important to educate people and to encourage public discussion about death and dying. Knowledge alone may be insufficient to change practice but education and discussion could be the first steps toward better palliative care provision for all in need.

5. Conclusions and implication for the future

In the future, the need for palliative care in the community will increase. Education about palliative care by *Last Aid courses* or other initiatives in combination with a compassionate community approach may serve to improve public discussion about death and dying, as well as palliative care provision in the community . There is a need for more research about *Last Aid courses* and other measures to empower the public to engage in palliative care provision in the community.

Possible conflict of interest

GB may have a potential conflict of interest as he receives financial compensation for teaching Last Aid Instructor courses. GB owns the trademarks "Last Aid" and "Letzte Hilfe".

Author details

Georg Bollig

1 Palliative Care Team, Medical Department Sønderborg/Tønder, South Jutland Hospital, Sønderborg, Denmark

2 Research Unit for Medicine and Palliative Care, Institute of Regional Health Research, University of Southern Denmark, Odense, Denmark

3 Last Aid International, Schleswig, Germany

*Address all correspondence to: georg.bollig@rsyd.dk

References

[1] Kellehear A. Compassionate communities: End-of-life care as everyone's responsibility. *The Quarterly Journal of Medicine*. 2013;**106**:1071-1075

[2] Kellehear A. Compassionate Cities. Public health and end-of-life care. Oxfordshire: Routledge; 2005

[3] Ewing G, Austin L, Jones D, Grande G. Who cares for the carers at hospital discharge at the end of life? A qualitative study of current practice in discharge planning and the potential value of using The Carer Support Needs Assessment Tool (CSNAT) approach. Palliative Medicine. 2018;**32**(5):939-949

[4] Etkind SN, Bone AE, Gomes B, Lovell N, Evans CJ, Higginson IJ, et al. How many people will need palliative care in 2040? Past trends, future projections and implications for services. BMC Medicine. 2017;**15**:102

[5] Bollig G, Gjengedal E, Rosland JH. They know! - Do they?: A qualitative study of residents and relatives views on advance care planning, end-of-life care, and decision-making in nursing homes. Palliative Medicine. 2016 May;**30**(5):456-470

[6] Seattle Fire Department. https://www.seattle.gov/fire/safety-and-community/medic-ii-cpr-training

[7] Bollig G. Palliative Care für alte und demente Menschen lernen und lehren. Berlin: LIT-Verlag; 2010 http://www.lit-verlag.de/isbn/3-643-90058-6

[8] Heller A, Wegleitner K. Palliative Care in der stationären Altenhilfe –Ansätze der Implementierung. In: Knipping C, editor. Lehrbuch Palliative Care. Bern: Hans Huber; 2006. pp. 73-80

[9] Heller A, Wegleitner K, Heimerl K. Palliative Care in der (stationären) Altenhilfe—Ansätze der Implementierung. In: Heller A, Heimerl K, Husebø S, editors. Wenn nichts mehr zu machen ist, ist noch viel zu tun. 3rd ed. Freiburg: Lambertus; 2007. pp. 351-366

[10] Bollig G, Kuklau N. Der *Letzte Hilfe* Kurs—ein Angebot zur Verbesserung der allgemeinen ambulanten Palliativversorgung durch Information und Befähigung von Bürgerinnen und Bürgern. *Z Palliativmed*. 2015;**16**:210-216

[11] Bollig G, Heller A. The last aid course - a simple and effective concept to teach the public about palliative care and to enhance the public discussion about death and dying. Austin Palliative Care. 2016;**1**(2):1010

[12] Bollig G. The Last Aid Course – Teaching the Public About Palliative Care. Lecture 21st International Congress on Palliative Care Montréal, Canada. Journal of Pain and Symptom Management. 2016. DOI: 10.1016/j.jpainsymman.2016.10.100

[13] Bollig G. The "Last Aid" course—an approach to promoting public discussion, awareness and education. SPPC Annual Conference 2017: Making the Best of Hard Times. Sep 2017. Edinburgh. https://www.youtube.com/watch?v=0mAAIXH2xPY

[14] Bollig G. What do people associate with the term "*Last Aid*"? In: Posterpresentation International Palliative Care Network Conference. 2018

[15] Bollig G, Brandt F, Ciurlionis M, Knopf B. Last Aid course. An education for all citizens and an ingredient of compassionate communities. Healthcare (Basel). Jan 28 2019;7(1)

[16] European Association for Palliative Care. Report and recommendations

of a workshop on palliative medicine education and training for doctors in Europe; 1993. www.eapcnet.org

[17] Partridge AH, Seah DS, King T, Leighl NB, Hauke R, Wollins DS, et al. Developing a service model that integrates palliative care throughout cancer care: The time is now. *Journal of Clinical Oncology*. 2014;**32**(29):3330-3336

[18] Singer PA, Wolfson M. The best places to die. BMJ. 2003;**327**:173-174

[19] Edwards SB, Olson K, Koop PM, Northcott HC. Patient and family caregiver decision making in the context of advanced cancer. *Cancer Nursing*. 2012;**35**(3):178-186

[20] Hudson P, Quinn K, Kristjanson L, Thomas T, Braithwaite M, Fisher J, et al. Evaluation of a psycho-educational group programme for family caregivers in home-based palliative care. *Palliative Medicine*. 2008;**22**(3):270-280

[21] Hudson P, Thomas T, Quinn K, Cockayne M, Braithwaite M. Teaching family carers about home-based palliative care: Final resulta from a group education program. *Journal of Pain and Symptom Management*. 2009;**38**(2):299-308

[22] Death Cafe. http://deathcafe.com

[23] Death chat. Talking about death and dying remains one of the biggest taboos within most communities. http://www.stchristophers.org.uk/social-programme/death-chat

[24] Preis der Deutschen Gesellschaft für Palliativmedizin. http://www.letztehilfe.info/auszeichnungen/preis-der-deutschen-gesellschaft-f%C3%BCr-palliativmedizin/

[25] Im Bundeskanzleramt/startsocial. http://www.letztehilfe.info/auszeichnungen/im-bundeskanzleramt-startsocial/

[26] Mueller E, Bollig G, Becker G, Boehlke C. Lessons learned from introducing "Last-Aid" courses at a university hospital in Germany. Abstract accepted for posterpresentation, 16th World Congress of the European Association for Palliative Care in Berlin, Germany; 2019

[27] Bollig G, Mainzer K, Fiedler H, Barra F, Pothmann RA. New Last Aid Course for Kids from 8-14 Years: A Pilot-test. Abstract accepted for posterpresentation, 16th World Congress of the European Association for Palliative Care in Berlin, Germany; 2019

[28] EAPC Taskforce Last Aid. Last Aid: Providing Palliative Care Education for Citizens. https://www.eapcnet.eu/eapc-groups/task-forces/last-aid

[29] Ferris FD, von Gunten CF, Emanuel LL. Knowledge: Insufficient for change. *Journal of Palliative Medicine*. 2001;**4**:145-147

Chapter 2

The Marquette Palliative Care System

Richard R. Love and Sheikh Iqbal Ahamed

Abstract

Worldwide, major clinical barriers to effective palliative care are the absence of a. current data on symptom type and intensity; b. immediately accessible information on practical, affordable, and effective interventions; and c. self-sustaining systems to facilitate physician engagement in continuing palliative care. Our adaptable system, developed for Bangladesh and Nepal, addresses these barriers. A tele-home palliative care program facilitates home care, minimizes expense, and encourages efficient professional practitioner involvement employing two information technology tools: a patient cell-phone "app" on the Android platform with a 15-item symptom questionnaire and an Internet website with health information sections for patients/families and for clinicians. The physician section contains a guide for patient symptom review, clinical practice palliative care guidelines, secured patient demographics, medical summaries, and current and past symptom reports along with prescription-writing capability. The system is managed by a local organization that registers patients and their physicians, instructs patients on the free downloadable application and completes their demographic and medical summaries, and arranges collection of a modest fee. The organization also ensures regular physician/clinic visits by the patient or by a family member with a patient phone check-in, at least every 2 weeks.

Keywords: palliative care, accessibility, symptom data, intervention information, efficiency, "app", tele-care, IT tools, home care, health

1. Introduction

1.1 Societal versus medical practice perspectives on improving palliative care

Reviews of country-by-country palliative care efforts, such as that provided by the Economist Quality of Death Index report, have identified broad area indicators of better palliative care, but such analyses ignore the weaknesses of prevailing clinical practice and health systems, which are poorly organized to provide patient-centered palliative care (**Table 1**) [1]. Ultimately, it is in clinical practice, the collective activities of health care providers, that the majority of critical activities bearing on actual patient palliative care experiences occur. To a great degree, the broad area indicators reviewed reflect community and political interest as well as financial investment. Unquestionably, such attention can, over time, lead to higher-quality palliative care, but throughout the world what governs the experience of individual patients needing palliation is primarily determined by the organization of medical practice, the attention of clinicians, and the focus of health systems. In the United States, as Emanuel has suggested in identifying key directions for the future of medical practice, effective organizations are those that transform provider interactions in palliative care [2]. It is in this context that the goals of this communication are addressed: more immediately than can occur to address the broad national and community indicators, how can general clinical practice globally be favorably affected to provide efficient and more effective palliative care for all patients needing such service? We describe here an information technology tool-facilitated basic system we believe is easily implemented and widely adaptable to clinical practice circumstances in many countries. By addressing common major barriers to provision of palliative care, we can increase practitioner engagement in such care at significant patient-benefiting levels.

1.2 Challenges and barriers to high-quality palliative care in clinical practice

Three-quarters of patients with advanced cancer are reported to suffer from pain and "85% of patients (with pain) can be well palliated with the use of simple, inexpensive, 'low technology' oral analgesics" [3, 4]. Unfortunately, however, there is little evidence supporting the long-term benefit of these analgesics and other symptom-alleviating interventions [5]. What and where are the barriers to closing these gaps? (**Table 2**).

A primary barrier to provision of adequate symptom treatment for patients is a clinical practice failure sequence: under-appreciation from under-assessment by clinicians of the types and intensities of symptoms patients are experiencing, which then logically is associated with very limited or absence of interventions to address these or the consequent helplessness and hopelessness that are root causes of suffering [4–6]. To provide optimal care for patients with cancer and other life-threatening illnesses, practitioner-available accurate, complete, and timely information about symptoms, daily information if possible, is necessary. Specifically, repeated failure among physicians worldwide to use validated symptom assessment tools prevents communication between patients and health-caregivers that could bring attention to symptom issues [7]. The usual way such information is obtained is through direct questioning or information provided in completing paper instruments during patients' relatively infrequent (and typically very brief) office visits with medical practitioners. If symptomatic status information could be obtained regularly, for example on a daily basis, and brought to the attention of the caring practitioners, this would be expected to improve symptom management and decrease suffering. This kind of activity is what characterizes comprehensive hospice programs and contributes significantly to their effectiveness for patients and their positive image for family members. Additionally, the development of regularly obtained symptom data would provide the basis for measuring, reporting, and improving the quality of palliative care, all absent in general current practice [2].

National policies addressing palliative care
Higher levels of public spending
Extensive training of health professionals
Patient care subsidies
Availability of opiate drugs
Public awareness

Table 1.
National indicators of higher quality palliative care. From 2015 quality of death index of the Economist [1].

Practitioners lack current patient data on symptom presence and severity
Practitioners lack practical, quickly accessed information on palliative interventions
Lack of efficient local systems for providing palliative care, particularly at home
Insufficient numbers of health professionals
Higher level interventions with no practical effect in the short- or medium-term, including increasing numbers of hospices, specialists, or specialist training activities

Table 2.
Barriers to effective palliative care in clinical practice.

A second major palliative care practice barrier is the absence of immediately-accessible information on locally practical, affordable, and effective interventions. A generally useful approach to more widespread use of effective interventions across the board in medicine has been the development and promotion of clinical practice guidelines. Academic approaches to such palliative care guidelines have been comprehensive, but overwhelming in their dimension and their lengths, and thus impractical for over-scheduled clinicians everywhere. The American NCCN clinical practice guidelines for palliative care are 106 pages in length [8]. Increasingly, attempts are underway to create succinct and practical palliative care clinical practice guidelines specific to each country to address all of the common symptoms, and that are well-grounded in local conditions and circumstances. There has been, however, even more limited attention to facilitating access to such guidelines and employment of their recommendations.

A third major palliative care practice barrier worldwide is the absence of efficient systems and processes to facilitate physicians' engagement in successful palliative care. Components of this situation are the understandable interest of patients and families in home care over institution or medical facility care, a dearth of practitioners in low- and middle-income countries comfortable with palliative care problem-solving and practice, and general clinical practice circumstances in which physicians are overburdened. Further, even if physicians were to have patient symptom and applicable intervention information readily available, their practice systems are not organized to allow them to provide home care as part of the workload for which they can be appropriately compensated financially. Worldwide, the palliative care manpower shortage situation cannot be realistically addressed by scaling-up training of adequate numbers of palliative care specialists. The practical approach is to facilitate engagement of physicians across all practice specialties in basic palliative care, under cost-effective and efficient locally-acceptable systems. The Economist investigation recognizes this need in emphasizing that training for all doctors and nurses is essential [1].

In general, there is a lack of approaches that consider whole populations in a public health perspective that addresses clinical-practice systems to provide for palliative care needs. Calls for increasing manpower of palliative care specialists, residential hospices, or educational activities regarding palliative care, even if successful, can simply not be expected to address adequately the large numbers of patients needing palliative care. These calls stem from the usual starting point—a provider-centric model of health care that needs to be replaced by a more patient-centric model. Simplistically speaking, the evolution of our health systems, particularly in the United States, has been grounded in addressing how things can and should ideally work for providers fixing problems, not supporting patients. This has led to organizational functioning and operations that produce fragmented care oriented to a disease; patient goals, wishes, perspectives and, most importantly, needs are regularly ignored. Addressing palliative care better can logically start by focusing on these patient-centered factors. In many ways, articulating an approach to palliative care is a tabula rasa, because, according to the Economist report documents, it is only in some high-income countries that apparently reasonable levels of palliative care for those in need are being provided [1]. Our personal experiences over the last 15 years in multiple health care settings across Asia, most particularly in Bangladesh (ranked 79 out of 80 countries in the Economist report), support the general conclusion that for the majority of global citizens, palliative care, at even the most basic levels, is nonexistent. It is within this broad perspective that the authors present the current innovations. Under the premise that information technology (IT) tools could contribute constructively to creation of patient-centered, effective, and cost-effective palliative care systems feasible within diverse health care systems in low- and middle-income countries (LMICs), we have been working for several years to develop practical, user-friendly, affordable IT tools and systems which address these afore-stated barriers [9–11].

2. A patient-centric, generalizable palliative care system that addresses common clinical practice barriers

2.1 Acquiring real-time symptom data: development of the patient questionnaire tool

If, instead of seeking paper questionnaire data on symptoms at the times of office visits, symptomatic status information could be obtained regularly on the day's experience from home by use of patient cell phones and delivered to attentive and responding physicians and caregivers in real-time in a well-organized way that complements prevailing overburdened physician practice with appropriate financial compensation, we could expect to improve symptom management and decrease suffering. Changing the collection and recording of patient symptom data from a medical staff task, currently done inefficiently and irregularly, if at all, to a patient task and responsibility has multiple major consequences [7]. First, it obviously simplifies and eases the operations of often hectic and overburdened clinic staff. In circumstances where electronic medical records have been extensively implemented, a well-described scenario occurs: the addition of more and more features makes the software system progressively more frustrating to use, developing it into what is called a "Tar Pit". Second, it allows creation of a legible standardized record of symptoms, which can be permanently filed in some patient record system. Simple standardization of a rating system enhances clinical staff interpretation of those records and easily notices and responds to a (sudden) increase in any one symptom. Third, critically, it engages the patients and their family members in openly identifying in detail the breadth of common symptoms. Fourth, and perhaps even more critically, the process of recording and submitting symptom reports by cell phone sets the stage for increased patient and family expectations about attention to those very symptoms.

Experienced clinicians report that when they have provided such means for patients to report specific data, expectations are high that there will be a closing of the loop with a clinician's response. In the circumstances of serious symptom report, for example a high level of pain, particularly if sudden and/or new, such empowered patients and family members react strongly if there are not prompt clinician responses. The perception is that if clinicians allow such information submission, they should have the capacity to process and act on it. The kinds of unhappy conversations that follow when patient reports do not elicit health professional or system responses can easily be imagined. In fact, when a patient computer-submitted report study that involved multiple practitioners did not train the practitioners beforehand in the creation of response systems, the clinicians experienced angry communications from patients and families in the absence of prompt responses to reports that demanded intervention. The practitioners quickly developed their own response systems to meet patient expectations, an example of a patient-driven change driven by enabling patients to communicate their needs.

We have first developed a basic cell phone symptom-status application, the reliability, feasibility, and validity of which we have established in studies in Bangladesh and Nepal [9–11]. The Marquette Symptom Assessment Survey (MSAS) is a 15-item questionnaire covering 12 symptoms; 4 items address pain dimensions. It is constructed using time-tested items from two well-validated and reliable instruments, the Edmonton Symptom Assessment Survey and the Brief Pain Inventory, and three additional items from prevailing palliative care practice: constipation, sleep quantity, and sleep quality [11–13] (**Table 3**). Current forms of this questionnaire in English, Bengali, or Nepali are presented on an Android cell-phone platform and display the questions in sequential fields in legible and audio-presented modes, allowing the patient, including those who are illiterate, to answer each question by moving a cursor along a Likert scale, which is a unidimensional 10-point visual analogue scale (**Figure 1**, top rating scale).

In a pilot study, 10 women with advanced breast cancer provided inter-rater and intra-rater reliabilities of >0.73, and patients or their caretakers were able to successfully submit reports despite progressive terminal illnesses [10]. These women and their families willingly and regularly submitted reports over several months. In <3 minutes, with minimal training, patients could and did answer the questions to indicate the presence and intensities of their symptoms. Subsequent extensive field testing and a large cross-sectional study of over 1000 patients with advanced cancers in Bangladesh and Nepal have established that this application is reliable, valid, and user-friendly, and can be employed by almost 100% of patients

Nausea[1]
Tiredness[1]
Depression[1]
Anxiety[1]
Drowsiness[1]
Appetite[1]
Well-being[1]
Shortness of breath[1]
Current pain[1]
In last 24 hours: worst level of pain[2]
lowest level of pain[2]
usual level of pain[2]
Constipation
Quantity of sleep
Quality of sleep

[1]*From the Edmonton Symptom Assessment Survey [12].*
[2]*From the Brief Pain Inventory [13].*

Table 3.
The Marquette Symptom Assessment Survey (MSAS).

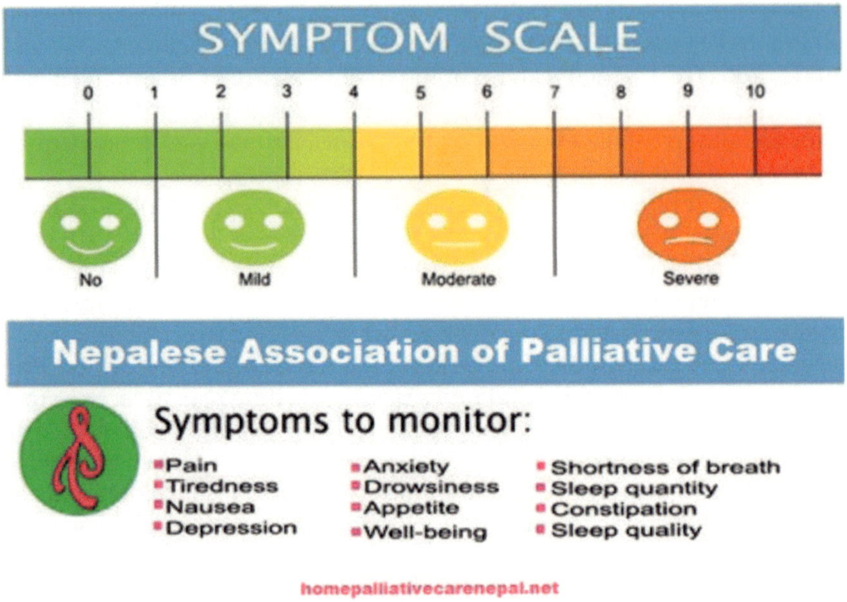

Figure 1.
Laminated symptom scale and symptoms-to monitor pocket ruler.

from a broad spectrum of socioeconomic circumstances. Specifically, in 640 adult Bangladeshi patients with advanced cancers under regular care in tertiary level institutions, all but two patients recruited agreed to study participation; all of these 638 patients had no trouble completing the questionnaire, despite the fact that some of the patients did not personally possess their own Android/smart phone [11, 14]. Only 2 patients out of the 640 said they would not choose to provide future monitoring data using this application [11]. Among 383 similarly recruited patients with advanced malignancies in Nepal, no patients refused study participation, all were able to complete the questionnaire rapidly, and none said they would refuse to provide future monitoring data with this questionnaire. Cell phone penetrance in Bangladesh is >90%; our Bangladeshi colleagues estimate that perhaps 50% of Dhaka residents have Android phones. In Nepal, more than 90% of families have access to cell phones, 2/3rds of which are estimated to be Android phones.

Assuming that patients can understand the symptom-intensity Likert scale and that there are no major cultural factors which influence specific patient reports such as language interpretations of the end-points, for example, or beliefs that there are "right" answers, which might lead to mid-scale scores, it is important to ask how we should define mild, moderate, and severe scores, and what unit changes in scores might be truly meaningful for patients. We have explored some of these cultural issues in our data from Bangladesh and have concluded that our data present a true picture of patients' symptoms [14]. With respect to word definitions in English for describing symptom intensity, we have chosen to consider as "mild" symptom scores of 3–4; otherwise our definitions are similar to those widely used. It is important to note that the scales are graphically as well as verbally defined. Regarding clinically significant score changes, for pain, it is reported that changes of 1–2 units, or down from moderate (5–6 score) to mild 1–4 scores, are, for patients, clinically significant [15].

In summary, we have developed a reliable and validated symptom assessment tool, specifically tailored to palliative care by adding questions about constipation and sleep because these issues are frequently of importance for such patients. This tool has been easily and rapidly used by essentially all studied patients (together over 1000) in two low-middle income countries. Importantly, ongoing repeated use was favorably perceived by patients and family members, even in the face of suboptimal patient symptom relief. After the deaths of relatives, family members repeatedly told staff members receiving the symptom reports how grateful they were for the opportunities to regularly engage the staff in assisting their loved ones. To them, often the most important matter was that everyone was paying attention to their relatives' symptoms. Thus, requesting and recording patient experience can be validated even when no intervention is possible—the opposite of clinician abandonment.

2.2 Using the MSAS to develop palliative care data on specific population symptoms to direct interventions

While the foregoing barrier considerations are all valid and should be the focus of interventions, successful palliative care management must begin with some understanding of the numbers, levels, and types of symptoms experienced by patients with limited life expectancy and the implications of that experience. Thus, we began as Cleeland did some 25 years ago in the United States, investigating the symptom picture for patients with advanced malignancy in two low- and middle-income country (LMIC) sites [11, 16]. The cross-sectional study described above allowed such evaluation for populations in Bangladesh and Nepal [11, 14, 17].

In Bangladesh, usual pain scores were ≥5 in two thirds of patients, but few patients had very high or minimal scores [11, 14]. Majorities of patients reported moderate scores for tiredness, nausea, depression, anxiety, drowsiness, poor appetite, and poor sleep [14]. The reported high intensity levels of these symptoms were not surprising to our Bangladeshi clinician colleagues. Collectively these symptoms contributed significantly to the suffering of these patients. For example, pain scores were correlated significantly with scores for nausea, anxiety, and poor sleep [14]. The patient population studied here might be expected to have a lesser symptom burden than that of the broad population of palliative care-needing patients in the country, because these patients were able to travel and seek care in tertiary care institutions. Overall, we interpret these data to suggest that there is high level and multi-symptom suffering among patients needing palliative care in Bangladesh, despite access to tertiary level care. The moderate pain scores for the majority of patients studied, along with minimal frequencies of high-score levels, suggest partial- and under-treatment. These conclusions are consistent with the Economist report assessment for the country, and with, for pain, the low level of narcotic consumption per capita [1, 18]. More important for the current communication is the practical usefulness of the tool used and these data in developing and targeting interventions [14]. Specifically, it is reasonable to suggest that under-treatment might be partially addressed by physicians having more symptom information in real time, the very issue our cell phone system seeks to address.

In Nepal, among the 383 studied patients, 37% reported maximal pain scores of 7 or greater [17]. Disturbingly, 5% of patients reported maximal pain scores of 10 [17]. A total of 59% of subjects however reported minimal pain. Again, the majority of patients reported moderate or greater levels of tiredness, depression, anxiety, poor appetite, and poor sleep. Alarmingly, 15% and 19%, respectively, reported severe depression and anxiety scores [17]. Our interpretation of these data is that again the cell phone questionnaire tool was very useful in developing reliable and informative data. Here, in contrast to Bangladesh, it appeared that a major fraction of the population had no pain management intervention at all.

In summary, in two LMIC settings, we have been able to demonstrate that our cell phone questionnaire tool can be used to develop important, clinically-useful patient symptom data.

2.3 Creating access to clinical practice guidelines

As discussed above, a practical barrier for clinicians to effectual palliative care is having easy and quick access to information about evidenced-based interventions. For LMIC settings, the first issue is creating such guidelines. Ideally, such guidelines would involve, as they have in high-income countries, comprehensive, rigorous, and transparent local processes involving a large cross section of local stake-holders and experts. The challenge, of course, is that such activities are expensive. Recognizing that the perfect is the enemy of the good, and that having some credible palliative care clinical practice guidelines in each of our pilot LMIC sites would be better than having none, we have created local guidelines in each country. Using the limited resources and experts available, we grounded these documents on local and international sources [8]. The 7-page document for Bangladesh is available at ag-palliativecare.net and the 13-page version for Nepal is available at HomepalliativecareNepal.net. Both were based on the outline presented in **Table 4**. Palliative care goals were informed by the understanding that "Survival is linked to symptom control, and pain management contributes to broad quality of life improvement [8]." Specific targets are to have as many as possible of the 12 common symptom scores in the mild range (4 or less) of the 10-point Likert scales and to lower moderate pain scores of 5 or 6 to at least a 4.

2.4 Coordinating information flow through a multi-user website

To integrate the cell phone questionnaire patient data and the clinical practice guidelines for practitioners in a system that will facilitate provision of palliative care interventions, we have created websites in Bangladesh and Nepal (ag-palliativecare.net and HomepalliativecareNepal.net). Patients submit their symptom questionnaire data to the website over the usual telephone systems. Each of these websites has six sections. There is an introductory home page that explains the system and a health information section for patients and their families. For all

• Palliative care goals
• General approach-psychological support
• Patient education
• Adult pain
• Sleep
• Poor appetite/constipation/feelings of unwellness/nausea
• Anxiety
• Depression
• Disclaimers
• Authors
• Accessible resources

Table 4.
Clinical Practice Palliative Care Guidelines.

participants, an “About us” section describes the operating organization and a contact information section provides a “hotline” telephone number. For health professionals, there is a general background informational section and a secure physician’s section accessed using user name and password, with further authorization for prescribing.

Entering this section, physicians can access the following:

- The Clinical Practice Palliative Care Guidelines.
- Basic descriptive instructions for patient symptom report review.
- A menu of types of the different reports that can be generated with one click.
- A list of specific patients registered to each clinician.
- Current or most recent MSAS reports for their patients.
- An historical graph of any score for last 14 or 28 days.
- Individual demographic and medical summary data for their patients, as outlined in **Tables 5** and **6**.
- A link to specific Clinical Practice Guideline intervention suggestions if any moderate or greater symptom score is reported.
- Twice-weekly alerts by text and/or email, by physician’s preference, if any patient reports symptoms with an increase in the level of an individual item score by more than 2 units, or a pain score of level 7 or greater results.
- A follow-up alert after a phone call has prompted a patient to send a confirmatory duplicate report to correct for patient entry errors.
- A prescription-writing field, with links to specific Clinical Practice Guideline intervention suggestions, and a menu of commonly prescribed drugs, standard indications, recommended doses, and standard use instructions. When an individual menu item is selected, drug, dose, and usage instructions automatically fill the individual patient’s prescription field. When the patients’ field is clicked on, their name and the date and other data required for prescriptions, as well as the physician’s name, are also automatically entered into the prescription field. A prescription cannot be completed without independent physician identity confirmation digital delivery is available.

2.5 Integrating the system with clinician and clinic practice

At least every 2 weeks, there will be a visit to the responsible physician. In recognition that repeated clinic visits may be a burden to family or patients, may worsen the very symptoms that are the target of care, and may even not be possible, the clinician will see either the patient or a family member. If the patient is not physically present at the clinic, the physician will call him or her during the visit, and confirm the information shared by a family member. This will also discreetly serve to avoid opioid theft and diversion, as well as to confirm that the patient is alive and receiving medication. Further benefit of the clinic visits

Name
Date of birth
National identity number
Home address
Patient mobile phone
Patient email address
Patient facial photograph
Family or closest friend contact information:
1. Name
Contact information
2. Name
Contact information
Notes:

Table 5.
Patient demographic dashboard.

Name
Major medical problems and diagnoses
Current major symptoms (most recent MSAS report)
Symptom MSAS score Date
Current medications (most recent prescription)
Notes:

Table 6.
Patient medical summary dashboard.

is continuity of record keeping, so that the palliative care website can remain auxiliary and does not need to match or duplicate any one facility's medical record system. These visits will also coordinate palliative care with the facility billing procedure, ensuring that physicians will be compensated at their usual rates for their time and expertise and encouraging their participation in the palliative care program. Palliative care is therefore insulated from the economic, administrative, and political concerns of a facility and does not interfere with the compensatory concerns of the physicians.

2.6 Engaging the Marquette Palliative Care System

Use of the cell phone symptom questionnaire "app" described in Section 2.1 and the website described in section 2.4 by physicians and patients is managed under the following system: patients or physicians contact the local system operating organization to learn about and register for system use. In Bangladesh, this is a nongovernmental organization, Amader Gram, and in Nepal, this organization is The Nepal Association for Palliative Care (NAPCare).

The local organization:

- Educates patients and families (and physicians) about the system. An essential requirement is that ongoing use of the system requires a clinic visit to the responsible physician at a maximum of every 14 days by the patient or a family member.

- Registers the patient and doctor in the website system so that cell-phone submitted patient symptom reports will be accepted and filed, associated with the responsible physician.

- Provides the physician with a website doctor's password and obtains a fingerprint for prescription writing verification/security.

- Provides the physician with a pocket-sized paper copy of the local Palliative Care Clinical Practice Guidelines as described in Section 2.3 and a laminated symptom-scale and symptoms-to-monitor pocket ruler (**Figure 1**).

- Encourages conduct of a baseline palliative care assessment clinical visit to clarify and codify breadth of patient medical diagnoses, specific symptoms and their likely pathophysiology, patient and family goals, and an overall palliative care plan (**Table 7**).

- Completes, along with the patient, the demographic "dashboard" database for that patient (**Table 5**) and identifies the responsible physician who agrees to provide care for that patient using the system.

- Works with the responsible physician using the baseline assessment data to create the medical summary "dashboard" database, and posts this database on the website.

- Assists patients in obtaining the cell-phone patient symptom questionnaire application from the Google store.

- Trains the patient and family in making symptom assessments, and then recording, and submitting them to the website.

- Arranges for payment (or waiving) of modest monthly fee to the local organization for submission of the reports and their availability on the system website. Use of an online payment system like PayPal can facilitate these transactions. Note that this fee can remain small because it covers the administration of the efficient palliative care system, not medical care compensation.

- Provides a text and telephone trouble-shooting "hotline" for patients and physicians and insures coverage.

- Maintains smooth operation, security, and accuracy of the website system. Reviews and updates the clinical practice guidelines periodically.

- Acts as an intermediary with responsible physicians for patient crises.

- Seeks feedback from the patient, families, and physicians regularly on system operations and problems and vigorously seeks to extend the use of the system, by marketing, to as large a patient population as possible.

- Seeks peer review of anonymized patient data and management for quality assurance to evaluate quality of care.

- Seeks to develop and conduct a rigorous evaluation of the entire system to determine the impact of the system on patients' symptoms, quality of life, and survival.

- Seeks, from the start-up phases on, to develop an operational business model that secures local system sustainability.

Date of evaluation:
All major medical diagnoses
(For cancer, list primary site of origin and sites of known clinical metastases)
1.
2.
3.
Performance status (ECOG scale 1–4)
Vital signs: Blood pressure, pulse, respiratory rate, temperature
Weight BMI
Height
Results of the most recent examination showing disease status:
Physical examination (+findings)
Imaging tests:
Hemoglobin
Current symptoms by Marquette Symptom Assessment Survey
Pain: Maximal pain score
Minimal pain score
Usual pain score
Current pain score
Major site(s) of pain and presumed causes (Inflammation, neuropathic, diffuse or focal bone, other)
MSAS score
Tiredness
Nausea
Depression
Anxiety
Drowsiness
Anorexia
Illness
Shortness of breath
Constipation
Sleep quantity
Sleep quality
Patient major goals
Family concerns and goals
Management plan
Problem/symptom Intervention/treatment

Table 7.
Palliative care baseline assessment checklist.

2.7 Piloting the Marquette Palliative Care System in Bangladesh and Nepal

In 2013–2014, the cross-sectional study described above was done in both Bangladesh and Nepal [11]. As detailed earlier in this chapter, considerable developmental work with the tools and on the system described here has been done in Bangladesh. By the end of 2017, the website and software had been developed and we were ready to launch the system as a business with Amader Gram. Unfortunately, various Amader Gram personnel and broad political uncertainty in the country have subsequently prevented further activities as of the end of 2018.

During the last half of 2018, we have been setting up the website and the operational system for this palliative care service model in Nepal. During the first 6 months of 2019, major clinical piloting experience with this system will be underway at a major cancer hospital outside of Kathmandu.

3. Implications and ideas for better global palliative care going forward

How to respond meaningfully to the data from reports like those of the Economist and to general calls for addressing palliative care globally is challenging [1, 19]. In this chapter, we argue that there can be a constructive way forward with immediate impact by taking a patient-centric, bottom-up approach to clinical practice systems, their barriers to palliative care, and the potential of IT tools and software. The system we present can in part and wholly be adapted to other country's circumstances, through a relatively minor investment of resources. High-income countries are beginning to develop and use such tools and systems in palliative care, and integration of such systems into established electronic medical record systems is achievable when the control issues can be worked out [2]. Until then, this system can economically function as a program auxiliary to facilities with medical records and those without. The system we present is particularly important in being directed at engaging clinicians/physicians who might otherwise avoid, refer, or somehow abandon their patients who now need palliative care. It can also be employed in noncancer specialties other than oncology that deal with chronic pain, and even be a resource for clinicians with less frequent need for palliation, or those in rural areas with fewer resources. Because our system is patient-centric and relies on and facilitates greater patient and family engagement and control, it also encourages stronger family support.

The entire system focus on palliative care might be expected to generally lower the total care costs, with minimal patient family expenses for submission of symptom reports and clinical office visits. In general, while limited, the available data suggest that facilitating home palliative care is effective for symptomatic relief of patients and is grief-limiting for families, while the overall cost efficacy remains to be well-understood [20]. We believe that after being extensively piloted, our system in Nepal and Bangladesh should be rigorously evaluated in a randomized clinical trial to document the impact on symptoms over time and overall patient survival.

The increasing use of IT technologies in patient care, including the use of video images and consultations, offer many ways of adding to the capacities of the system we describe. It would very much seem that affordable, efficient, and effective home care/palliative care should be within the reach of many more countries and global citizens.

Acknowledgements

The authors wish to acknowledge very helpful discussions about the development of the system discussed in this chapter with Reza Salim, Tahmina Ferdousy, Arunangshu Das, Bishnu Paudel, Deepak Shrestha, and Roshni Gautam.

Author details

Richard R. Love* and Sheikh Iqbal Ahamed
Department of Mathematics, Statistics, and Computer Science, Marquette University, Milwaukee, Wisconsin, USA

*Address all correspondence to: richardibcrf@gmail.com

References

[1] Economist Intelligence Unit. The 2015 Quality of Death Index. London: The Economist; 2015

[2] Emanuel EJ. Prescription for the Future: The Twelve Transformational Practices of Highly Effective Medical Organizations. Public Affairs. New York: Perseus Books; 2017

[3] Twycross RC, Fairfield S. Pain in far-advanced cancer. Pain. 1982;**14**:303-310

[4] Grossman SA, Nesbit S. Cancer Pain in Clinical Oncology, 3rd Edition, Abellof MD, et al., eds. Philadelphia: Elsevier; 2004. pp. 715-730

[5] Ballantyne JC, Sullivan MD. Intensity of chronic pain—The wrong metric? The New England Journal of Medicine. 2015;**373**:2098-2099

[6] Cassel EJ. The nature of suffering and the goals of medicine. The New England Journal of Medicine. 1982;**306**:639-645

[7] Au E, Loprinzi CL, Dhodaptkar M, et al. Regular use of verbal pain scale improves the understanding of oncology inpatient pain intensity. Journal of Clinical Oncology. 1994;**12**:2751-2755

[8] https://www.nccn.org/professionals/physician_gls/pdf/palliative.pdf [Accessed: 05-11-2018]

[9] Kawsar FA, Haque MM, Adibuzzaman M, et al. e-ESAS: Improving Quality of Life for Breast Cancer Patients in Developing Countries. MobileHealth@MobiHoc. 2012. pp. 9-14

[10] Haque MM, Kawsar FA, Adibuzzaman M, et al. Findings of mobile based palliative care system: Towards formulating a generic framework for measuring QoL. In: 8th International Conference on Pervasive Computing Technologies for Healthcare; 20-23 May 2014; Oldenburg, Germany. Brussels: ICST; 2014. pp. 1-8. DOI: 10.4108/icst.pervasivehealth.2014.254960

[11] Love RR, Ferdousy T, Paudel BD, et al. Symptom levels in care-seeking Bangladeshi and Nepalese adults with advanced cancer. The Journal of Global Oncology. 2016;**3**:257-260. DOI: 10.1200/JGO.2016.004119

[12] Bruera E, Kuehn N, Miller MJ, et al. The Edmonton symptom assessment system (ESAS): A simple method for the assessment of palliative care patients. Journal of Palliative Care. 1991;**7**:6-9

[13] Cleeland CS, Ryan KM. Pain assessment: Global use of the Brief Pain Inventory. Annals of the Academy of Medicine, Singapore. 1994;**23**:129-138

[14] Love RR, Ahsan GMT, Ferdousy T, et al. Symptoms in Bangladeshi patients with incurable cancers: Implications for interventions. Indian Journal of Palliative Care. 2018;**24**(2):173-175

[15] Serlin RC, Mednoza TR, Nakamura Y, et al. When is cancer pain mild, moderate or severe? Grading pain severity by its interference with function. Pain. 1995;**61**:277-284

[16] Cleeland CS, Gonin R, Hatfield AK, et al. Pain and its treatment in outpatients with metastatic cancer. The New England Journal of Medicine. 1994;**330**:592-596

[17] Love RR, Paudel BD, Ahsan GMT, Ahamed SI. Symptoms in Nepali Patients with incurable cancers: Implications for interventions. (Submitted to The National Association of Medical Sciences Postgraduate Journal)

[18] University of Wisconsin-Madison: Pain & Policy Studies Group. http://www.painpolicy.wisc.edu/countryprofiles

[19] Knaul FM, Farmer PE, Krakauer EL, et al. Alleviating the access abyss in palliative care and pain relief-an imperative of universal health coverage: The Lancet Commission report. Lancet. 2018;**391**:1391-1454. DOI: 10.1016/S0140-6736(17)32513-8

[20] Gomes B, Calanzani N, Curiale V, et al. Effectiveness and cost-effectiveness of home palliative care services for adults with advanced illness and their caregivers. Cochrane Database of Systematic Reviews. 2013;**2013**(6):CD007760-CD007760. DOI: 10.1002/14651858.CD007760.pub2

Chapter 3

Palliative Care Ethics: Medicine's Duty to Help

Sukru Keles

Abstract

In palliative care, death, which is a part of human nature, is considered as a normal process. This type of care is concerned with the quality of life rather than its duration. In this context, the basic aim is to perform practices to relieve the patient in a way that does not raise any ethical suspicion. Within this framework, it can be said that palliative care is a requirement of medicine's duty to help. The aim of this chapter is to draw attention to the importance of ethical values in the configuration of palliative care services for patients who are in the last period of their life or the ones who have terminal illnesses. In palliative care, it is essential to arrange care services in a manner that does not raise any ethical doubt about the measures taken to increase beneficence both to the patients who are in the last days of their life and to their relatives. In this study, "The Directive for Implementing Procedures of Palliative Care Services" prepared by the Ministry of Health in Turkey in 2015 will be evaluated in terms of ethics.

Keywords: bioethics, medical ethics, clinical ethics, palliative care ethics, directive

1. Introduction

Ethics is a branch of medicine that deals with the questions as to the values such as "What's good" or "What's good for people" [1]. Medical ethics is a branch of general ethics which centers on moral issues encountered in the field of health. In this respect, medical ethics is a field where the emerging moral issues, particularly the ones stemming from the medical advances witnessed in the twenty-first century in diagnosis and treatment tools, are discussed.

In health ethics, studies on the evaluation of moral priorities in the field of health and in legal, political, or institutional aspects and the analysis of their possible outcomes have been carried out. Different from medical ethics, health ethics deal with issues that concern a larger majority of the society. Ethical evaluation of health decisions made on a societal level and in accordance with the regulated norms, policies at hand, and supported projects is one of the topics of interests in health ethics.

The right to a healthy life is a fundamental human right. Everyone has the right to receive healthcare, and this right is guaranteed by the constitutions of nations. The right to healthcare is a positive right. Therefore, healthcare providers are expected to create opportunities for the beneficiaries. Besides, configuration of different kinds of health services in healthcare is essential.

There is a close relation between health ethics and the legal regulations for maintaining healthcare services. The significant point in terms of health ethics is that the legal regulations are drawn in an ethically acceptable manner. In this respect, "The Directive for Implementing Procedures of Palliative Care Services" prepared by the Ministry of Health in Turkey in 2015 will be evaluated in terms of ethics in the subsequent sections of the study [2]. With that directive, it was aimed to provide medical, psychological, social, and moral support to both patients and their relatives when life-threatening diseases are at stake. It can be said that the Directive, which comprises basic ethical principles and their extensions, satisfies the expectations of patients and their relatives from palliative care services to a large extent [3].

Given that the organization of palliative care services across the country is a recent trend, it can be envisaged that palliative care will be accepted by healthcare demanders as an accessible and claimable healthcare service in the forthcoming years.

2. Palliative care and "confidence" in medicine

In the literature of medical ethics and philosophy, the necessity to perform certain actions or deeming them as necessary is considered to be a "duty" [1]. The duty of a healthcare professional or a physician is based on carrying out an action that she/he is authorized or allowed to do in an appropriate manner. In established philosophical thinking, at least from Kantian thinking to modern philosophy, the concept of duty in ethics means acting from intention without any compulsion and believing that it is the right thing. As a requirement of social contract, the sense of duty forms the basis of behaving ethically. In this respect, regardless of any legal and juridical imposition, healthcare professionals feel themselves responsible for the practices they perform and act accordingly and provide healthcare services to patients. It is imperative that healthcare professionals carry out their duties in accordance with the medicine's raison d'être in order to maintain the confidence in medicine.

Healthcare professionals are expected to care for patients and be sensitive to their needs. The thing to consider here is paying regard to beneficence to the patient and helping the patient improve his/her current condition. A relationship based on trust between the healthcare professional and the patient or the patient's relatives is a prerequisite to pursue the implementation of healthcare services at the optimum level. Providing healthcare services to anyone who requests it is one of the most fundamental duties of healthcare professionals.

Palliative care is not centered solely on patients; it also covers the practices such as fulfilling the needs of patients' relatives as well. This includes helping the patient's relatives in the mourning days, after the loss of the patient. Palliative care service is carried out by a team, and each step of the process is accompanied by healthcare professionals qualified in their field.

The World Health Organization (WHO) defines palliative care as follows:

"Palliative care is an approach that improves the quality of life of patients and their families facing the problem associated with life-threatening illness, through the prevention and relief of suffering by means of early identification and impeccable assessment and treatment of pain and other problems, physical, psychosocial and spiritual" [4].

The emerging points in the definition of the WHO are:

i. Palliative care ethics focuses on moral problems related with the end of life.

ii. Patient care shall not be defined just with medical procedures; social, cultural, economic, and belief systems are also the important components.

iii. Human is a creature who must be respected; therefore, the quality of death should be equally esteemed as the quality of life.

In societies where the philosophy of palliative care is not fully comprehended, such care practices are frequently confused with other practices. It should be noted that palliative care is not:

i. Letting the patient to die

ii. Assisting the patient to die

iii. Speeding up the patient's death

iv. Sustaining the life in an artificial manner

The quality of palliative care is closely related to "confidence" in medicine. In order to provide palliative care to a patient in the last days of his/her life, it's imperative that the patient demands this care at his/her own request and approves of it. The patient should be informed about the purpose of palliative care and the possible benefits of it. It is crucial that the patient has competence to give such a decision and approve of the procedure. Within the context of medical ethics, competence means an individual's ability to make autonomous decisions concerning his/her own health [1]. When a competent individual whose life is coming to an end loses his/her competence, he/she must have unconditional confidence in medicine as to what kind of healthcare he/she will receive. It is disputable how to act in conditions where competence is lost due to the cultural values in different societies. Therefore, the most ethically appropriate act would be taking into account the decision that the patient made when he/she was still competent and assuring the patient in this regard when she/he had competence.

3. Palliative care and the patient's "compelling" medical condition

Recently, a number of opinions have been generated as to the fact that care services to be provided for life-threatening diseases shall not be limited to medical theories and practices and that the related culture, economy, society, and political environment must also be taken into account [5, 6]. In palliative care, life-threatening diseases are needed to be handled with a holistic approach, and for this reason, a care service performed by a multidisciplinary team is offered to patients and their relatives. In palliative care, ethical values specific to this "challenging" period are emphasized, and suggestions for resolving ethical problems are debated [7, 8].

Contemporary palliative care began at the end of the 1950s by means of observing dying patients and providing healthcare services to them. Dr. Cicely Saunders observed dying patients and stated that an interdisciplinary team could be able to alleviate the pain of dying patients and their relatives. Today, providing end-of-life care with a team of healthcare professionals constitutes the core of palliative care services. Dr. Elisabeth Kübler-Ross, who was a psychiatrist in the USA in the 1960s, emphasized in her book *On Death and Dying* the importance of open, respectful, and honest communication with dying patients. In 1974, Dr. Balfour Mount pointed out the importance of a holistic approach in respect of physical, mental, and social aspects to patients who have life-limiting illnesses and their families. In 1997, with the report "Approaching Death: Improving Care at the End of Life," the Institute of Medicine documented the shortcomings related with the end-of-life care and paved the way for a growing interest in palliative care in medical practices. In addition, "Clinical Practice Guidelines for Quality Palliative Care" was published in 2004, and since then palliative care services have been offered to not only dying patients but also the ones with life-limiting diseases [9].

Today, palliative care is given to patients from various age groups and for different illnesses. The difficult conditions in which the dying patients or patients with chronical diseases and their relatives go through might cause health professionals to feel themselves desperate in providing healthcare to them, just like a family mourning for their child would feel [10]. It was reported that when the risk of losing a family member emerges, it influences all members negatively [11]. A previous study emphasized the importance of giving the families reliable and comprehensible information during those challenging times. In that study, it was also pointed out that the technical information which medicine offers is not sufficient and must be reinforced with emotional care, which is also an important aspect [12]. In addition, it was emphasized that communication skills and ethical professional values still constitute the essence of medical practices despite the increasing use of advanced technologies and increased information in the field of health [13]. Paying regard to the humanistic side of medicine in the delivery of palliative care services to patients and their relatives is possible only when health professionals develop an ethical sensibility and have ethical conscience.

Hospices constitute an alternative to hospital-centered care. The purpose of hospice care is to provide an effective pain treatment in order to bring symptoms such as nausea, vomiting, diarrhea, and weight loss under control and to relieve the patient through nutritional and ventilatory support. It is different from conventional hospitals in that its priority is, within the bounds of resources available, to help dying patients and their relatives before their lives come to an end. These days, the interest in hospices is increasing due to the aging population, and this brings about ethical problems. The most notable ones among the problems encountered in hospices include upholding resident autonomy, managing family distress, lack of staff communication, and lack of time [14]. It is clear that providing healthcare services in hospices with an approach that pays regard to the values of patients and their relatives will increase the confidence in these newly developed health centers.

4. Proliferation of palliative care practices in Turkey

According to Tanrıverdi and Kömürcü, studies on structuring palliative care services in Turkey started with the initiatives of the Society of Algology, which was founded by Dr. Serdar Erdine, an anesthesiologist and reanimation specialist, in 1998, and the early studies carried out on pain palliation [15]. In the same period, medical oncologist Dr. Şeref Kömürcü studied the concept of palliative care in oncology. Following these initiatives, "Supportive Treatments Study Group" was established in 1999 within the body of the Turkish Society of Oncology Group. The Cancer Dispensary, which was established in Turkey by Turkish Oncology Foundation and actively served between the years 1993 and 1997, is considered to be the first institution that is close to the concept of hospice where palliative care services are offered [16, 17]. This was followed by the establishment of Ankara House in 2006 by Hacettepe University Cancer Institute. The Ankara House, also referred to as "Hacettepe House of Hope" is a hospice that offers palliative care services and treatment and accommodation to cancer patients for a certain period of time. However, the House could not actively serve for a long time.

One of the reasons why proliferation of hospices in Turkey is a more recent process than in Western counties is believed to be the prevailing negative perceptions of the society on the concept of retirement home for old people, which has become a privatized healthcare service for the last decades [17]. In today's world, proliferation and improving the quality of healthcare institutions such as home care services, retirement homes, and nursing and rehabilitation centers for old persons reinforce the confidence in social aid and social service works.

Palliative care services have become more widespread through the project "Palya-Turk" conducted by the Cancer Control Department of the Ministry of Health. Nevertheless, when the existing need for palliative care in Turkey is considered, it can be said that the current palliative care services fail to fully meet this need [18]. Besides, it has been pointed out that the palliative care provided in Turkey for patients with chronical diseases or the ones close to the end of life is perceived as a care service offered only to cancer patients [19]. However, it is acknowledged that the primary issues to be dealt with are building a trust relationship between health professionals and patients and their relatives, enabling active participation of patients and their families to decision-making processes and improving the patients' quality of life by means of avoiding futile treatments [20]. Today, palliative care services are provided, though on a limited level, either at home or at health institutions depending on the type of illness.

4.1 The palliative care directive in Turkey and the emerging ethical values

"The Directive for Implementing Procedures of Palliative Care Services," which regulates the minimum standards of palliative care centers founded within the body of inpatient health institutions, was put into effect with the regulatory dated June 07, 2015 and numbered 253 [2].

In these centers, patients can receive various healthcare services including physical examination, medical work-up, analysis, treatment, medical care and rehabilitation services, psychosocial support, psychosocial evaluation (distress, anxiety, depression, hope, loss, mourning, grief, and self-care), pain management (opioid use), nutritional support, and so on. In addition, the centers can also issue medical reports as to a patient's need for medication, medical devices, and medical equipment.

The abovementioned Directive constitutes the framework for delivery of palliative care in Turkey. The backbone of the Directive is to improve patients' and their relatives' quality of life in order to alleviate or prevent their pain and suffering [3].

First section

Objective, Scope, Basis and Definitions

> *Article 1—"The objective of this Directive is to enable early identification and assessment of pain and other symptoms of patients occurring due to life-threatening illnesses, to alleviate or prevent pain by providing medical, psychological, social and moral support to these persons and their family members, to establish palliative care centers with the aim of improving their quality of life, and to determine the rules and procedures as to these centers' operation, physical conditions, minimum standards for equipment and personnel, duties and responsibilities of the personnel, and supervision of their practices."*

Quality of life: some of the opportunities that modern medicine offers contribute to lengthening life-span. Palliative care aims to increase the quality of life. The meaning content of the quality of life is one of the topics that are being discussed by moralists and philosophers [21]. Also, one of the questions that awaits answering in terms of ethics is what gives value to human life. In this respect, the value of life is considered together with the quality of life. Improving the patient's physical and emotional well-being within the bounds of possibility in order to improve the quality of life is one of the raisons d'être of palliative care. In this way, it is aimed that the patient shall continue his life, make choices, and maintain communication with his environment as much as possible.

A person's life is important not only to himself but also to his family members, friends, acquaintances, and other people with whom he/she has an emotional relationship. Therefore, in palliative care, the cordial relationship that the patient establishes with his/her relatives and the well-being of the individuals apart from the patient are also taken into consideration. In this respect, one of the most important constituents of the Directive is that it enables patients to spend time with their relatives in an appropriate environment.

Besides, the Directive also aims to standardize the centers that provide palliative care in order to improve the life quality of the patients struggling with life-threatening diseases. This has stemmed from the intention to help structuring healthcare services in a sense that they are accessible and claimable and to bring a common perspective to the palliative care philosophy.

Second section

Establishment of centers, physical conditions and minimum standards for equipment, provision of transportation vehicles

Article 5—(1) "Palliative care services are provided at palliative care centers in inpatient care institutions, home care service units outside those institutions, and family practice centers. Impatient care institutions can make a protocol with care centers for giving palliative care to the ones staying there and provide palliative care service on condition that it is ratified by the Directorate."

Proliferation of palliative care: palliative care services are provided in various types of health institutions in order to make it a more widespread and common practice. Palliative care centers in Turkey are organized as (i) "primary level" palliative care centers that encompass palliative care units at family practice centers and hospitals, (ii) "secondary level" that includes palliative care centers (acute care), and (iii) "tertiary level" which covers comprehensive palliative care centers (acute care) and hospices (chronic care) [22]. In this way, a patient can benefit from a variety of palliative care units that best suit their needs.

Article 6—(1) "The number of beds at a palliative care center to be established within the body of a health institution shall not exceed 25% of the total number of beds for a hospital with 100 or less beds, 20% for a hospital with 101-300 beds, 17% for a hospital with 301-500 beds, and 15% for a hospital with 501 or more beds."

A fair resource allocation: the fact that the minimum number of beds in hospitals to be used for palliative care has been determined through the Directive brings up the issue about how to share the limited resources in an ethically appropriate manner. The question as to which criteria should be taken into account while evaluating the patients requesting this care is ethically disputable because different point of views on allocation of limited resources may lead to different practices. In this respect, subjective considerations can also be evaluated such as the patient's medical condition, prognosis of the illness, the amount of time that the patient need palliative care, and the beneficence of palliative care to the patient and his/her relatives. In the Directive, there is no information about how to allocate beds among patients. However, this could be a deliberate preference because it might have been deemed inappropriate to determine the selection of patients to benefit from this care with the Directive since it is a patient-specific process confined to the patient's unique conditions.

In addition, receiving consultancy service from ethical committees for accepting patients to the centers with limited patient admission capacity should be fostered since this will save the responsible physicians from making the decision alone.

> *Article 6—(2) "Procedure and Examination Rooms are the places equipped with appropriate medical equipment and devices where physicians can intervene to their patients and where family negotiations and services such as psychological and social services shall be provided. When necessary, an appropriate number of procedure and examination rooms can be designated. Occupational Room is an optional facility where patients receive physical therapy, occupational therapy, speech and language therapy, treatments and services to relieve them physically and psychologically, and where family negotiations and psychosocial services are provided."*

Privacy: the presence of special areas in which the healthcare staff who provide palliative care services deal with the needs of the patients and their relatives is an indicator of respect for their private lives. In addition, the presence of occupational rooms might help reduce the challenging factors that patients and their relatives encounter during this period. The presence of unwanted people during an intervention or examination might violate privacy. In this context, paying regard to the necessary spatial arrangements for the provision of a humanly end-of-life care to the patient and for the protection of the patient's relatives from being disturbed can be considered as an indicator of ethical sensibility.

All kinds of information that the physician get in patient-physician relationship is dealt within the scope of professional confidentiality [23]. In this respect, the Directive could also entail that physicians shall not reveal patients' secrets or confidential information that they obtain from the encounters with patients. It is acknowledged that this liability of the physician should continue after the patient's death or termination of the patient-physician relationship.

The Directive can be given as an example to the practices that reduce the patient load of the intensive care units where life-supporting treatments are performed and to the places where procedure and examination rooms are prepared for patients requesting palliative care when needed. Such practices can facilitate the access to treatment needs of other patients in the hospitals. In the literature, it was argued that when the patients requiring palliative care occupy beds in hospitals for a long time, it reduces the efficiency of the facilities offered in those hospitals [24].

> *Article 7—(1-2) "Transportation and transfer vehicles allocated for health institutions and directorates that offer home care services can be used by the centers as well if necessary. (...) In case of emergency, patients shall be transferred via the ambulances of health institutions or 112 emergency services."*

Patient transfer: it is possible that patients might get harmed during their transfer to healthcare centers or to another city. In the Directive, it was stated that patients' transfer might be assisted if necessary and that it is tried to prevent the damages to occur due to the transfer process. The attempt to avoid any risks toward a patient before they emerge reflects the existence of a sensibility in line with the medicine's ethical principle of non-maleficence.

Third section

Personnel assignment and minimum personnel standards, duty, authority and responsibilities

> *Article 8—(1-5) "(...) The services at the center shall be performed under the responsibility of the physician in charge along with the other personnel including physicians, nurses, medical secretary, administrative and technical staff, cleaning staff and so on. (...) There's no obligation to recruit a full-time psychologist, social worker, physical therapist or physical therapy technician, and dietician at the center, but if any need emerges, it shall be met by the hospital's own staff or from external sources. (...) Necessary training of the staff recruited for palliative care services in the centers shall be provided by the Administrator."*

Duty of education: in palliative care, the responsibility of identifying and solving the problems of patients and their relatives is expected primarily from those who provide that service at the outset. Allowing patients and their relatives to express themselves and facilitating communication might prevent any harm that may occur to them to a large extent. Therefore, along with their residency training in palliative care, it is also important to offer education on basic ethical knowledge, including trainings on communication skills and problem-solving methods for persons who provide palliative care services.

The trainings given to healthcare professionals in order to improve the quality of service should also cover the issue of identifying the ethical problems faced in palliative care. Therefore, training of the staff that is in charge of providing palliative care for patients with chronical diseases or the ones close to the end of life could eliminate the mistakes to be made out of ignorance. However, it is crucial to reinforce ethical knowledge education since it puts healthcare professionals who has benefited from this training in a situation where they confront their own values. It is obvious that provision of ethical education for those who provide palliative care services will contribute to building the ethical standards in palliative care.

Fourth section

Working Principles and the Scope of Service

> *Article 11—(1-4) "The centers assess the palliative care provided to patients and family members as a whole and take all kinds of necessary precautions with a team mentality in order to ensure that they get the most out of the service. (...) Under the coordination of Provincial Directorate of Health, the centers aim to raise public awareness on palliative care by means of collaborating with local governments, other health institutions in the region, universities and other related organizations, and if necessary, visual and print media."*

Biopsychosocial model: being aware that the patients and their relatives have their own universe of values shall increase the quality of the palliative care services offered. Therefore, it should be accepted that patients and their relatives have different health needs. Being aware of the values and belief systems of the patients and their relatives; assessing each patient as a whole in respect of physical, psychological, and social aspects; and taking precautions accordingly are the conducts all of which should be supported ethically.

Ethics of health education: during monitoring and observation processes, healthcare professionals working at the centers contribute to improving the patients', their relatives', and, indirectly, the society's health. The healthcare professional responsible for training and preserving the holistic approach of the profession plays an active role in patients' and their relatives' decision-making processes through active participation. Health educators carrying out works on raising people's awareness must consider the differences in the structure of society as a value and act accordingly.

Fifth section

Application for Palliative Care Services, Patient Admission, Transfer and Transportation Principles

Article 13—(1) "Applications shall be made in person by the patients themselves or by their family members, or they shall be directed to the center or the healthcare provider who provides palliative care services after necessary consultation and coordination has been made during the patient's discharge by means of maintaining necessary negotiation and coordination with the curative doctor or family practitioner who is in charge of the patient's follow-up and treatment. Through a visit by a health team, the patients who are unable to come to a health facility shall be assessed in their home environment as a whole, along with the family members that they live together. As a result of the assessment, the patients found eligible to receive palliative care service shall be referred to the centers."

Paternalism: in palliative care, it may be on the carpet that, for the sake of protecting their patients fighting against life-threatening diseases or to relieve their distresses, the physicians in charge might adopt a paternalistic approach based on their sensibility they have developed for the individuals in this group. However, in contemporary way of ethical thinking, it is ethically troubling for a physician to make decisions in lieu of the patient without any reasonable ground. Therefore, interventions made without the consent of the patients or their relatives might be interpreted as violation of personal rights.

Seeing the patient and the patient's relatives by the responsible physician both in the palliative care center and in the patient's house has several advantages. Encouraging the patient to make an autonomous decision and listening to the patients and their relatives without governing them are ethically appropriate attitudes and behaviors.

Time: in palliative care, "time" is a special component of limited resources. Beginning to provide palliative care services at the right time for a patient who is at the last period of his/her life is this service's reason for being. According to the Directive, enabling the patients who are found eligible for palliative care to benefit from this opportunity "just because they need it" is an ethical responsibility.

Article 15—(1-3) "The centers determine the palliative care patients residing within their service area by means of making use of the records that family practitioners and home care service units keep, and then create their own database. (…) It is obligatory to take the necessary security precautions in order to record separate files for each patient, to record register and follow-up books, to record data in computer environment and to protect them in the period and manner as specified in the legislation, and to share personal and statistical information of the patient."

Protection of personal data: in the Directive, protection of the personal data of the patients is deemed obligatory. Personal data comprise information about an individual's identity and also include information as to a patient's illnesses. The principle of non-maleficence to the confidentiality of the patients and their relatives entails respect for their private life. Members of the team providing palliative care services can share patients' personal or statistical data with the second or third parties or with the relevant institutions only to an extent that the patients permit. In the contrary cases, it can be stated that the individual's private life is not respected, and this means that respect for autonomy, which is one of the basic ethical principles, is violated. Therefore, such practices are ethically unacceptable.

Sixth section

Patient Rights, Termination of Service, Training, Supervision and Responsibility

Article 16—(1) "Patients accepted to palliative care services shall be informed about patient rights and liabilities and the content of the service. The patient himself or his legal representative has the right to receive all kinds of information about the service to be provided and the risks (if any). And, the patient has the right to refuse the service. Legislation provisions regarding patient rights are reserved."

Informing the patient and the patient's volunteering: it can be seen that the Directive respects persons and pays attention to patient autonomy. The patient's volunteering for admission to palliative care is regarded as a value in line with the principle of respect for patient's autonomy. The patient's volunteering is based on the information given to the patient as to the content of palliative care service. Therefore, in the Directive, a special attention was attached to informing the patient. The basic reason for emphasizing its importance is to ensure that the patient rights, which are part of human rights specific to the field of medicine, are reflected on medicine in practice. Otherwise, the patient's volunteering might be at risk, and the patient's autonomy might be damaged. Giving incomplete information to the patient about the end-of-life or his/her chronical diseases, pressuring the patient, and deceiving the patient about the possible benefits of palliative care might impair the patient's volunteering; therefore, such practices are ethically unacceptable. In the delivery of palliative care services, healthcare professionals are expected to ensure that patients receive a care service compatible with human dignity in the challenging conditions they face. Moreover, the patients' giving of consent for the palliative care to be offered to them is based on the information given to them and making sure that it was fully comprehended by them. At this stage, the content of the information to be given to the patients demanding palliative care or their relatives is important. The understanding of what palliative care constitutes the "informing" phase of the process. Also referred to as "getting informed consent," the process is the reflection of the basic ethical principle of respect for autonomy on the field of medicine.

Refusal to healthcare: in line with the principle of respect for autonomy, healthcare professionals who provide palliative care services should understand it when a patient refuses to receive care service on his/her own consent. Therefore, they should neither force patients or their families to receive palliative care services nor put pressure on patients in order to persuade them. The most ethically appropriate approach would be letting the patients make their own decisions as to the healthcare services they will receive no matter how big their pain and suffering is.

Article 17—1 (b) "In the event that the patient's or his legal representatives demand termination of the service, or that the patient or his family members exhibit misbehavior and resist to comply with the recommendations, the beneficence of the service is questioned by the specialist physician in charge, and the decision regarding the termination of the service shall be made by means of negotiating with the patient and family members, and the decision shall be recorded with an official report."

Terminating the care: it cannot be claimed that palliative care fits for its purpose if the patient does not benefit from the provided service. According to the Directive, if no positive change is observed in respect of the patient's quality of life, a decision to terminate the service shall be made. Such a decision cannot be made by the physician alone. In the Directive, it was pointed out that the patient or patient's relatives should also be included in the decision-making process for termination of palliative care. Besides, if the patient claims that she/he has benefited from the treatment psychologically, though not physiologically, the physician's termination of care service is not ethically appropriate. Palliative care can be terminated if patients or their relatives consider palliative care as unnecessary or there is strong evidence that the planned care does not make a positive contribution to the patient's quality of life.

5. Conclusion

As well as the principles that it recognizes, medicine is also renowned for the practices that it deems unacceptable on ethical grounds. Practices such as overlooking the health needs of patients with chronical diseases or terminal patients and disregarding their healthcare needs, for instance, are ethically unacceptable.

The conditions that patients or their relatives face might sometimes hinder them from pursuing a quality life. If they prefer, they can receive palliative care, which can give them a chance to have a fairly quality life. Palliative care is crucial for maintaining the confidence in medicine and cannot be considered separately from the medicine's duty to help.

In Turkey, how and by whom palliative care should be given to a patient approaching to the end of his/her life is determined by the relevant directive. Providing the service in line with the legislation and regarding patient rights, professional ethics, and medical deontology is essential. In palliative care centers, under the coordination of Provincial Directorate of Health, health services are provided in collaboration with local authorities, other health institutions in the region, universities, and with other related institutions. Besides, the centers also take the responsibility to contribute to the training of the society by means of planning trainings that go beyond the institution.

The fact that the Directive involves the doctrine of informed consent, which is the reflection of the principle of respect for autonomy on medical practices, illustrates the importance attached to patient rights in palliative care services. Nevertheless, there are still issues to be dealt with such as identifying the ethical dilemmas, which may emerge due to telling the patients and their relatives the truth, giving them the bad news, and decision-making for the end-of-life decisions, and taking measures in order to solve them. Ethical mistakes that healthcare professional make out of ignorance might be eliminated if their knowledge on the issues not covered in the Directive is reinforced through in-service trainings.

Early identification and assessment of life-limiting diseases match up with the raison d'être of palliative care services. In this context, palliative care aims to support both the patients and their family members who encounter such problems when it comes to life-threatening diseases. In order to identify the ethical problems seen in palliative care services in Turkey, qualitative and quantitative studies are needed to be carried out. As palliative care services become a more common practice in Turkey and more sophisticated solutions are offered as to the ethical problems encountered in practice, the structure of the palliative care service delivery will also go through transformation.

Conflict of interest

The author declares that there is no conflict of interest regarding the publication of this article.

Other declarations

This chapter is an expanded version of the article published in the Supplement Issue of Journal of Anesthesia (JARSS) with the title "Palliative Care Services Directive and Ethical Values" (see Şükrü Keleş, "Palliative Care Services Directive and Ethical Values". Journal of Anesthesia (JARSS). Supplement. 2017, 25(3):15–19).

Author details

Sukru Keles
Department of History of Medicine and Ethics, Hacettepe University Faculty of Medicine, Ankara, Turkey

*Address all correspondence to: kelesukru@gmail.com

References

[1] Oğuz NY, Tepe H, Örnek Buken N, Kırımsoy KD. Bioethics Glossary. Ankara: Philosophical Society of Turkey; 2005

[2] Republic of Turkey, Ministry of Health. The Directive for Implementing Procedures of Palliative Care Services. Available from: http://hizmetstandartlari.saglik.gov.tr/Eklenti/2817,palyatif-bakim-hizmetleri [Accessed: 2019-01-10]

[3] Keleş Ş. Palliative care services directive and ethical values. Journal of Anesthesia-JARSS. 2017;**25**(Suppl 3):e15-e19

[4] World Health Organization. WHO Definition of Palliative Care. Available from: http://www.who.int/cancer/palliative/definition/en/ [Accessed: 2019-01-20]

[5] Lewis MJ. Medicine and Care of the Dying: A Modern History. Oxford University Press; 2007. DOI: 10.1093/acprof:oso/9780195175486.003.0005

[6] Clark D, Graham F. Evolution and change in palliative care around the world. Medicine. 2011;**39**(11):636-638

[7] Lars S, Ulla M, Inger B. Developing organisational ethics in palliative care: A three-level approach. Nursing Ethics. 2017;**24**(2):138-150

[8] Bardach SH, Dunn EJ, Stein JC. Clinician perspectives on challenges to patient centered care at the end of life. Journal of Applied Gerontology. 2017;**36**(4):401-415

[9] Matthew JL. Palliative care: An historical perspective, ASH education book. Hematology. American Society of Hematology. Education Program. 2008:465. DOI: 10.1182/asheducation-2008.1.465. Available from: http://asheducationbook.hematologylibrary.org/content/2008/1/465.full

[10] Weaver MS, Lichtenthal WG, Larson K, Wiener L. How I approach expressing condolences and longitudinal remembering to a family after the death of a child. Pediatric Blood & Cancer. 2019;**66**(2):e27489. DOI: 10.1002/pbc.27489

[11] Davidson JE, Aslakson RA, Long AC, Puntillo KA, Kross EK, Hart J, et al. Guidelines for family-centered care in the neonatal, pediatric, and adult ICU. Critical Care Medicine. 2017;**45**(1):103-128. DOI: 10.1097/CCM.0000000000002169

[12] Ågård AS, Hofhuis JGM, Koopmans M, Gerritsen RT, Spronk PE, Engelberg RA, et al. Identifying improvement opportunities for patient- and family-centered care in the ICU: Using qualitative methods to understand family perspectives. Journal of Critical Care, ISSN: 1557-8615. 2019;**49**: 33-37. DOI: 10.1016/j.jcrc.2018.10.008 0883-9441/

[13] Büken Örnek N. Physician-patient communication during the clinical ethical decision-making process in palliative care in Turkey. Journal of Anesthesia-JARSS. 2017;**25**(Suppl 3):e3-e14

[14] Muldrew DHL, Kaasalainen S, McLaughlin D, Brazil K. Ethical issues in nursing home palliative care: A cross-national survey. BMJ Supportive & Palliative Care. 2018. ISSN: 2045-4368. BMJ Publishing Group; PMID: 30563824

[15] Tanrıverdi Ö, Kömürcü Ş. Palyatif Bakım Ünitelerinde Yapılanma. In: Gülhan M, Yılmaz Ü, editors. Akciğer Kanserinde Destek Tedavisi. TÜSAD Eğitim Kitapları Serisi. Probiz Ltd. Şti. 2016. pp. 391-407. e-ISBN: 978-605-66161-1-2

[16] Madencioğlu Kıvanç M. Palliative care services in Turkey. HSP. 2017,

2017;**4**(2):132-135. DOI: 10.17681/hsp-dergisi.316894

[17] Sur, H. Tıbben bitmiş sayılan ömürlere hospis çözüm mü? Sağlık Düşüncesi ve Tıp Kültürü Platformu. Available from: http://www.sdplatform.com/Yazilar/Kose-Yazilari/420/Tibben-bitmis-sayilan-omurlere-hospis-cozum-mu.aspx [Accessed: 2019-01-14]

[18] Şahan Uslu F, Terzioğlu F. Palliative care education and organization in the world and Turkey. Cumhuriyet Nursing Journal. 2015;**4**(2):81-90

[19] Demir M. Palliative care ethics. Yoğun Bakım Derg. 2016;7:62-66. DOI: 10.5152/dcbybd.2016.1202

[20] Akpınar A, Alvur M. Ethical and medicolegal issues in palliative care. Turkiye Klinikleri Journal of Family Medicine—Special Topics. 2017;**8**(4):292-298

[21] Boddington P, Podpadec T. Measuring quality of life in theory and practice. Bioethics. 1992;**6**(3):201-207

[22] Republic of Turkey, Ministry of Health General Directorate of Treatment Services, Health Services Planning in Turkey. 2011-2023. Available from: https://khgmsaglikhizmetleridb.saglik.gov.tr/TR,42884/turkiyede-ozellikli-planlama-gerektiren-saglik-hizmetleri-2011-2023.html [Accessed: 2019-01-09]

[23] Turkish Medical Association. Declaration of Respect for Private life. 2010. Available from: https://www.ttb.org.tr/kutuphane/etik_bldgeler2010.pdf [Accessed: 2019-01-23]

[24] Kabalak AA, Öztürk H, Çağıl H. End of life care organization; palliative care. Yoğun Bakım Dergisi. 2013;**11**(2):56-70

Chapter 4

Communication with Families in the Last Days of a Patient's Life and Optimal Delivery of a Death Pronouncement

Soichiro Okamoto, Yu Uneno, Masanori Mori,
Takashi Yamaguchi and Nobuhisa Nakajima

Abstract

Communicating with family members is critically important when a severely ill patient is experiencing their last few days of life. However, healthcare professionals (HCPs) have limited opportunities to learn effective and respectful ways to perform this communication. In recent decades, significant effort has been put forth to identify the phenomena that indicate the last hours and days of life and the optimal methods to deliver a death pronouncement, which will potentially help HCPs communicate compassionately with family members throughout the dying process. In this chapter, we will review the literature regarding the phenomena that indicate the last hours and days of life and the death pronouncement. Furthermore, we will discuss clinical implications derived from those articles and future research perspectives.

Keywords: communication, impending death, bereaving family, death pronouncement

1. Introduction

The death and dying of a loved one can place a serious emotional burden on his/her family members [1]. The methods of communication during the dying process and the death pronouncement are critically important because they can affect the families' acute emotional responses and their long-term psychological well-being [2]. However, there are limited opportunities to learn effective and respectful methods of how to communicate at the end of life and the pronouncement of a patient's death even though healthcare professionals (HCPs) often experience such challenges in daily practice.

Over the last decade, cumulative evidence has revealed various phenomena that indicate the patient is experiencing their last hours and days of life (e.g., death rattle, cyanoses, or Cheyne-Stokes respiration) [3, 4]. Sharing these bedside clinical signs with families can allow them to understand the patients' condition, estimate prognosis, and prepare for the impending event. Moreover, a recent unique research study regarding the death pronouncement (e.g., a video-vignette study design) revealed effective and respectful ways to deliver this pronouncement [5].

The communication processes between HCPs and family members can potentially reduce the unpleasant emotional responses of the families.

In this chapter, we will review the reported literature regarding communication during the dying process and death pronouncement. Furthermore, we will discuss clinical implications derived from those articles and future research perspectives.

2. Phenomena indicating the last hours and days of life

As the time of death approaches, patients with advanced cancer follow various clinical courses and commonly experience serious burdens such as pain, dyspnea, or delirium [4, 6]. Previous literature has reported that patients and their family members hope to be free from physical and emotional distress at the end of life, and it is challenging for HCPs to assess the patients' distress and deliver optimal care during end-of-life situations [7]. Understanding the bedside trajectory of the patients' symptoms and distress will potentially allow HCPs to develop a reasonable end-of-life care pathway, which enables them to share the patient's condition and promotes family members to prepare for the impending event [3, 8]. Actually, leaflet-based interventions that describe physical impending death signs have been revealed to improve family members' knowledge and distress throughout the dying process [9, 10].

We herein review the literature regarding representative and common phenomena that indicate the last hours and days of life.

2.1 Common symptoms in the last weeks of life

During the last 2 weeks of life, dyspnea, pain, increased bronchial secretions, and confusion occur with prevalence of 56.7, 52.4, 51.4, and 50.1%, respectively [4]. As death approaches, the prevalence of dyspnea and confusion increases [8]. Meanwhile, pain was reported to reach a stable level of intensity [8]. Thus, HCPs must not underestimate those common symptoms and other hidden signs of distress and symptoms in patients.

Accordingly, performance status also deteriorates throughout the dying process [8, 11]. Because of muscle weakness and refractory cachexia, time spent in bed increases. Moreover, patients experience difficulties with performing daily activities such as changing clothes, bathing, swallowing, etc. At this point, because of the loss of autonomy, patients often feel emotionally and spiritually burdened, and supportive communication to cope with these distresses must be encouraged.

2.2 Common symptoms in the last days of life

In 2013, a Delphi method study including a panel of palliative care experts reached a consensus that the following seven clinical signs serve as impending death signs: changing breathing rhythm and patterns (e.g., Cheyne-Stokes respiration, apnea), irreversible deterioration of consciousness, no fluid or food intake, marble-like skin, changing emotional status (e.g., restlessness, agitation), rapid degradation of general condition, and intuition of professionals (gut feeling) [12]. A unique longitudinal observational study revealed a detailed symptom trajectory in the last days of life [13]. In this study, apnea, Cheyne-Stokes respiration, increased bronchial secretions, dysphasia of liquids, a decreased level of consciousness, a palliative performance scale score $\leq$ 20%, peripheral cyanosis, pulselessness of the radial artery, respiration with mandibulae movement, and decreased urine output were recognized as impending death signs. Particularly, a palliative performance scale score $\leq$ 20%, decreased levels of consciousness, and dysphasia of liquids commonly occur in the last 3 days of life. The authors suggested dividing impending death signs into two categories: early and late signs [13]. Early signs (e.g., decreased performance status, decreased oral intake, and decreased level of consciousness) are observed relatively frequently. Because of their low specificity, these signs are not reliable predictive markers of a death event within 3 days. By contrast, late signs emerge only in the last few days of life in a smaller proportion of patients and had a high positive likelihood ratio for impending death within 3 days. The author concluded that late physical signs may assist clinicians in making a diagnosis of impending death [13]. The same research groups reported an inability to close the eyelids, drooping of the nasolabial fold, hyperextension of the neck, and grunting of vocal cords as promising impending death signs [14].

2.3 Detailed discussion of common symptoms and clinical signs

2.3.1 Pain

Pain control is a common clinical challenge at any stage of disease [15]. Pain in the last 2 weeks of life and 48 hours before death occurs with a prevalence of 44 and 54%, respectively [4, 7]. With inappropriate pain control, both patients and caregivers are likely to complain of fatigue, anorexia, and insomnia [16].

Various agents have been investigated to relieve cancer pain and pathophysiological assessments of pain (e.g., nociceptive, somatic, and visceral pain); therefore, selecting a reasonable treatment strategy is essential [17–21]. During the end-of-life stage, many patients suffer from swallowing difficulties, and in such cases, HCPs must consider alternative routes for administering analgesics to achieve appropriate pain control without interruption. Intravenous and subcutaneous administrations are stable, less invasive methods [22].

2.3.2 Dyspnea

Dyspnea results from several causes, including atelectasis due to tumor growth, pleural effusion, superior vena cava syndrome, pulmonary embolism, anemia, etc. [15, 23, 24]. The prevalence of dyspnea in the last 2 weeks of life is 56.7% [4]. Patient dyspnea is well known to be associated with family members' distress [25].

The effect of morphine on alleviating dyspnea has been well investigated [26]. Because of the deteriorated capacity of drug metabolism and excretory abilities during the end-of-life period, the administration of morphine requires careful monitoring of adverse events (e.g., impaired conscious state and decreased respiration rate) [26]. Given the concerns of those adverse events, physicians are less confident with prescribing opioids for dyspnea than for pain, which can result in the undertreatment of dyspnea [27]. Optimal clinical training is warranted in this setting. In addition, benzodiazepines can be a treatment option against refractory dyspnea [25].

In addition to pharmacological treatment, some non-pharmacological approaches are also promising for dyspnea. Recently, a unique study revealed that fan therapy toward the face is effective for patients with advanced lung cancer [28, 29]. Moreover, it is empirically known that changing body posture and discharging sputum are also effective methods of dyspnea care.

2.3.3 Increased bronchial secretions

With impending death, a rattle sound can be heard during both the inspiratory and expiratory phases around the upper respiratory tract area. Bennett divided this symptom into two subtypes: type I and II [30]. Type I is mainly caused by the accumulation of salivary secretions due to a decrease in consciousness and swallowing reflex [30]. Generally, anticholinergic drugs that suppress secretions from the salivary glands and endobronchial mucous are promising strategies to treat type I. Since type II is believed to be caused by purulent sputum such as tumor-derived secretions and pneumonia, anticholinergics are considered ineffective [30].

Classical anticholinergic drugs such as atropine, scopolamine hydrobromide, and glycopyrronium, which reduce secretions from the salivary glands and bronchial mucosa, are commonly used [31]. These medications can be administered sublingually, subcutaneously, and intravenously. Despite the cumulative experience of administering classical anticholinergic drugs among HCPs, there is a lack of sufficient investigations on their effects. A double-blinded clinical trial from Germany showed the superior efficacy of glycopyrronium compared to scopolamine hydrobromide [32]. In a randomized controlled trial conducted in Belgium, the subcutaneous administration of atropine, scopolamine butylbromide, and scopolamine hydrobromide showed an improvement of approximately 40% on a pre-post basis; no significant difference between the drugs was reported [33]. Recently, the prophylactic administration of hyoscine butylbromide was shown to effectively prevent the death rattle [34]. However, because a randomized controlled study found that atropine was not superior to a placebo control, anticholinergic drugs are not widely recognized as the gold standard treatment [35].

Since the rattle sound due to increased bronchial secretions may cause family members to anticipate patient distress, appropriate information sharing among family members and HCPs is crucial [36]. A survey for bereaved family members revealed that 66% felt distress due to the rattle sound and 53% reported the need to improve this symptom [36]. Conversely, another study found that the death rattle may not be associated with respiratory distress in coma patients [37]. In cases of refractory rattle sounds, HCPs must explain to family members that the patients are experiencing limited distress, and HCPs should continue care for their grief and suffering [37].

2.3.4 Delirium

Delirium at the terminal stage is occasionally described as agitation or terminal restlessness, which occurs as an irreversible symptom due to organ dysfunction [38]. Delirium occurred in 44% of patients during the last 7 days of life, and 88% of cancer patients with delirium had incurable end-stage delirium [38]. Delirium not only causes patients unbearable distress, but more than half (54%) of the family members reported distress as well [39].

To treat a patient's delirium, the reversible causes must be examined and treated (e.g., infection, electrolyte abnormalities, nutritional deficiency, dehydration, and medications). The administration of olanzapine, quetiapine, and aripiprazole may provide some benefits for the patient [40]. Although a clinical study showed that neither oral haloperidol nor risperidone had a demonstrable benefit on the symptomatic management of mild-to-moderate delirium, antipsychiatry drugs including haloperidol and chlorpromazine are generally used for delirium in end-stage patients [41, 42]. Administering haloperidol with lorazepam may benefit terminal cancer patients (median overall survival of 73 hours) with agitated delirium [43]. Since these drugs can be administered intravenously, subcutaneously, or intramuscularly, suitable administration is possible even in end-of-life patients. However, since it may fail to show improvements despite appropriate treatment and care, delirium is one of the most common reasons for the decision to initiate sedative therapy (57.1%) [44].

2.3.5 Vital signs

Vital signs include the level of consciousness, blood pressure, pulse rate, respiratory rate, O_2 saturation, etc. [45]. Vital signs are indicators that can reflect several abnormal and altered states of human biological status [46]. These indicators can often be surrogate markers of distress such as pain or dyspnea, even in patients with loss of consciousness. However, vital signs may have a limited role as prognosis predictors. Previous literature has revealed that blood pressure and O_2 saturation tend to decrease and body temperature tends to increase in the last 3 days of life, but their sensitivity and specificity to predict death within 3 days were 30 and 80%, respectively [45]. Thus, routine monitoring of vital signs may not be essential in end-of-life clinical practice.

2.3.6 Other clinical signs

Patients with Cheyne-Stokes respiration display abnormal respiration patterns that repeat cycles of apnea and a gradually increasing and decreasing respiratory rate [13]. During the last 3 days of life, 41% of patients experience this symptom [47].

Respiration with mandibulae movement is known as a late impending death sign. Patients unintentionally move their lower jaw up and down, commonly with loss of consciousness [13]. During the last 3 days of life, 56% of patients experience this symptom, which may predict death occurrence within 7.6 (±2.5) hours [48].

Cyanosis is caused by increased deoxyhemoglobin within the peripheral tissue. Central cyanosis is commonly derived from shock status and congestive heart failure, whereas peripheral cyanosis commonly affects local lesions caused by peripheral vascular disease [13]. At the end of life, cyanosis is believed to be caused by contraction of the peripheral vessels. During the last 3 days of life, 56% of patients experience this symptom, which can predict death occurrence within 5.1 (±1.0) hours [48].

2.3.7 Prognosis prediction

Prognosis prediction is also a critical issue in end-of-life care and is partially composed of the abovementioned symptoms and clinical signs. Several user-friendly clinical tools have been developed in previous studies, such as the palliative prognostic score, the palliative prognostic index, and prognostic in palliative care study predictor models [49–51]. Detailed discussion regarding this topic is described elsewhere [52].

3. Death pronouncement

When a patient dies, physicians must relay this information to his/her family members. Generally, to diagnose the patient's death, physicians examine the vanished pulse, respiratory cycles, and heart sounds [53]. This procedure is not only a clinical practice but is also a valuable opportunity for compassionate communication with his/her family members and can help alleviate their grief and emotional burden [53, 54]. Recent evidence has disclosed the optimal way to deliver a death pronouncement. However, the death pronouncement can be a considerably stressful event even for physicians, which potentially leads to unfavorable outcomes such as insomnia, anxiety, or depression. Brown et al. revealed that the death pronouncement can cause serious distress even in simulation settings [55]. Education for HCPs and healthcare students may play an essential role in coping with this distress. To date, several educational activities regarding death pronouncement and procedure guides have been developed.

We herein review the previous literature regarding the optimal method of delivering the death pronouncement and education on this topic.

3.1 History of death pronouncement education

Initially, narrative guidelines for death pronouncements were proposed in the early 1990s. In 1992, Terri A. Schmidt et al. proposed a program that included 17 recommendations on how to conduct interactions with survivors following a patient's sudden death in the emergency department [56]. This program required 2 1/2 hours to complete and allowed residents to practice their communication skills in a protected setting [56]. In the same year, the Office of Attorney General of Iowa proposed a recommended procedure for the death pronouncement called "in person, in time." This recommendation conveyed the following five concepts: "in person" (respect for privacy and for free emotional reactions), "in time" (information should be delivered as soon as possible), "in pairs" (news should be delivered by a team of two notifiers), "in plain language" (the message should be relayed directly; the notifier ought to speak slowly and in single sentences, giving details and answering questions), and "with compassion" (empathy, the attempt to understand emotions accompanying individuals who are notified about the death of a close relative, is essential) [57]. In 1998, Lucille Marchand et al. introduced brief clinical tips for residents, which included six steps (the phone call, the patient floor, in the room, the pronouncement, documentation, and when to call the corner), to clarify how the death pronouncement process should proceed [58].

3.2 Educational intervention regarding the death pronouncement

In conjunction with those narrative approach efforts mentioned above, the efficacy of the educational intervention was investigated. Marc et al. reported that one and a half lectures regarding the death pronouncement improved the skills of resident physicians who attended an ACLS course [59]. Lucille Marchand et al. reported on outcomes derived from a workshop based on six essential competencies (patient care, medical knowledge, practice-based learning and improvement, systems-based practice, professionalism, and interpersonal skills communication) proposed by the Accreditation Council for Graduate Medical Education's Outcome Project [60]. This workshop provided the opportunities to learn poetry, prose, and narratives on delivering death pronouncements by senior residents; reviews and discussion of protocols for death pronouncement, autopsy, and organ donation; and a roleplay of a death pronouncement with the opportunity for reflection [60]. In 2005, Bailey et al. examined the effectiveness of a 10-minute death pronouncement module and pocket-card guideline approach [54]. This intervention improved five self-assessed competencies, including three procedure skills (clinical examination for pronouncing death, writing the death note, and completing the death certificate) and two communication skills (informing the family about the death and assessing/managing family bereavement) [54]. In 2008, Hobgood et al. investigated the efficacy of a 2-hour teaching module based on the mnemonic "The GRIE_VING," which included small group discussion, roleplay, and didactic experiences [61]. This module improved resident confidence and competency scores on a pre-post basis [61]. The authors also reported on the efficacy of this intervention in fourth-year medical students [62]. In 2011, Nordstrom et al. reported a unique approach employing a marathon death exercise. This exercise was designed to enable fourth-year medical students to gain insight into the emotional and formal procedure of delivering a death pronouncement [63].

As mentioned above, a considerable number of studies that used lectures and/or roleplay for pre/post medical education showed promising efficacy.

3.3 Optimal method of delivering the death pronouncement

In addition to considering and discussing the optimal way to deliver a death pronouncement among HCPs, it may be helpful to acquire opinions from viewpoints of family members, which potentially include definite answers. Kusakabe et al. performed a survey of bereaved family members [64]. The families experienced a death pronouncement in home care settings, and 89% reported that there were no deficiencies throughout the process [64]. Family members reported that positive physician behaviors included acting calmly (not rushed), having a suitable appearance for the situation, introducing themselves to the family members, explaining the cause of death explicitly, and conducting a check using a light and stethoscope for the death pronouncement. Negative behaviors included a lack of clearly verifying the time of death and leaving the patient's clothes disheveled. Interestingly, Japanese family members did not appreciate touching the family members' backs or shoulders as an expression of empathy [64]. Hatano et al. also conducted a survey of bereaved family members from hospice or palliative care unit settings [65]. Overall, 86% of bereaved caregivers reported satisfaction with physician behavior toward the death pronouncement; however, 22% felt there were several areas requiring improvement. The bereaved caregivers did not appreciate automatic or routine pronouncement behaviors. Likewise, a logistic regression analysis revealed that "polite behavior" and the "physician introduced himself/herself to the family" were preferred behaviors. Confirmation by the primary responsible physician was significantly preferred than that by an unfamiliar physician [65]. Based on these findings of optimal behaviors, Mori et al. performed a unique study applying a randomized, scripted, video-vignette study design [5]. In this randomized, video-vignette study, volunteer participants viewed two videos of death pronouncements by an on-call physician with or without compassion-enhanced behaviors [5]. This behavior included five components: "waiting until the families calm themselves down, explaining that the physician has received a sign-out containing information of the patient's condition, performing the examination respectfully, ascertaining the time of death with a wristwatch (vs. a smartphone), and reassuring the families that the patient did not experience pain." Participants who viewed the compassion-enhanced behaviors video assigned significantly higher scores for physician compassion and trust in the physician and lower scores for anger, sadness, fear, and disgust. This study proposed recommendations that physicians should initiate a prompt examination, explain that they have received a sign-out, perform the examination respectfully, ascertain the time of death with a wristwatch, and reassure the families that the patient did not experience pain [5].

3.4 Future perspectives

As described above, several educational intervention models have been developed, and reasonable methods of delivering the death pronouncement have been proposed. However, one study suggested that only 35% of the procedures were judged as acceptable [66]. We must continue to grasp and improve the overall quality of the death pronouncement delivery by HCPs. Moreover, to determine the HCPs' burden in this setting, a scale that measures the difficulties of delivering a death pronouncement must be developed.

The next steps must investigate whether those interventions or behaviors truly improve the outcomes of bereaved family members (e.g., depression, anxiety, or substance abuse.) Accordingly, investigating the efficacy of alleviating the emotional burden of HCPs is also necessary. Continuous efforts to develop effective educational interventions and implement practical models that can meet the needs of several medical contexts are also warranted.

4. Conclusions

In this chapter, we narratively reviewed various phenomena that indicate the impending last hours and days of life and the death pronouncement within a scientific context. These findings can help enable HCPs to engage in compassionate communication with the family members who share the same ultimate goals. Further efforts to integrate and enhance this knowledge and these activities are warranted to alleviate the burden and distress of patients, family members, and HCPs.

Acknowledgements

This work was supported by JSPS KAKENHI Grant Number JP18K15396.

Conflict of interest

No conflicts of interest are declared.

Author details

Soichiro Okamoto[1], Yu Uneno[2*], Masanori Mori[3], Takashi Yamaguchi[4] and Nobuhisa Nakajima[5]

1 Asoka Vihara Hospital, Kyoto, Japan

2 Seirei Hospice, Seirei Mikatahara General Hospital, Shizuoka, Japan

3 Palliative Care Team, Seirei Mikataraha General Hospital, Shizuoka, Japan

4 Division of Palliative Care, Department of Medicine, Konan Hospital, Japan

5 Division of Community-based Medicine and Primary Care, University of the Ryukyus Hospital, Okinawa, Japan

*Address all correspondence to: yuuneno@kuhp.kyoto-u.ac.jp

References

[1] Krawczyk M, Gallagher R. Communicating prognostic uncertainty in potential end-of-life contexts: Experiences of family members. BMC Palliative Care. 2016;**15**:59

[2] Steinhauser KE, Christakis NA, Clipp EC, McNeilly M, McIntyre L, Tulsky JA. Factors considered important at the end of life by patients, family, physicians, and other care providers. Journal of the American Medical Association. 2000;**284**(19):2476-2482

[3] Seow H, Barbera L, Sutradhar R, Howell D, Dudgeon D, Atzema C, et al. Trajectory of performance status and symptom scores for patients with cancer during the last six months of life. Journal of Clinical Oncology: Official Journal of the American Society of Clinical Oncology. 2011;**29**(9):1151-1158

[4] Kehl KA, Kowalkowski JA. A systematic review of the prevalence of signs of impending death and symptoms in the last 2 weeks of life. American Journal of Hospice and Palliative Medicine. 2013;**30**(6):601-616

[5] Mori M, Fujimori M, Hamano J, Naito AS, Morita T. Which physicians' behaviors on death pronouncement affect family-perceived physician compassion? A randomized, scripted, video-vignette study. Journal of Pain and Symptom Management. 2018;**55**(2):189-97.e4

[6] de la Cruz M, Noguera A, San Miguel-Arregui MT, Williams J, Chisholm G, Bruera E. Delirium, agitation, and symptom distress within the final seven days of life among cancer patients receiving hospice care. Palliative & Supportive Care. 2015;**13**(2):211-216

[7] Ellershaw J, Smith C, Overill S, Walker SE, Aldridge J. Care of the dying: Setting standards for symptom control in the last 48 hours of life. Journal of Pain and Symptom Management. 2001;**21**(1):12-17

[8] Mercadante S, Casuccio A, Fulfaro F. The course of symptom frequency and intensity in advanced cancer patients followed at home. Journal of Pain and Symptom Management. 2000;**20**(2):104-112

[9] Otani H, Morita T, Uno S, Yamamoto R, Hirose H, Matsubara T, et al. Effect of leaflet-based intervention on family members of terminally ill patients with cancer having delirium: Historical control study. American Journal of Hospice and Palliative Medicine. 2014;**31**(3):322-326

[10] Otani H, Morita T, Uno S, Yamamoto R, Hirose H, Matsubara T, et al. Usefulness of the leaflet-based intervention for family members of terminally ill cancer patients with delirium. Journal of Palliative Medicine. 2013;**16**(4):419-422

[11] Hui D, dos Santos R, Chisholm GB, Bruera E. Symptom expression in the last seven days of life among cancer patients admitted to acute palliative care units. Journal of Pain and Symptom Management. 2015;**50**(4):488-494

[12] Domeisen Benedetti F, Ostgathe C, Clark J, Costantini M, Daud ML, Grossenbacher-Gschwend B, et al. International palliative care experts' view on phenomena indicating the last hours and days of life. Supportive Care in Cancer: Official Journal of the Multinational Association of Supportive Care in Cancer. 2013;**21**(6):1509-1517

[13] Hui D, dos Santos R, Chisholm G, Bansal S, Silva TB, Kilgore K, et al. Clinical signs of impending death in cancer patients. The Oncologist. 2014;**19**(6):681-687

[14] Hui D, Dos Santos R, Chisholm G, Bansal S, Souza Crovador C, Bruera E. Bedside clinical signs associated with impending death in patients with advanced cancer: Preliminary findings of a prospective, longitudinal cohort study. Cancer. 2015;**121**(6):960-967

[15] Teunissen SC, Wesker W, Kruitwagen C, de Haes HC, Voest EE, de Graeff A. Symptom prevalence in patients with incurable cancer: A systematic review. Journal of Pain and Symptom Management. 2007;**34**(1):94-104

[16] Ovayolu O, Ovayolu N, Aytac S, Serce S, Sevinc A. Pain in cancer patients: Pain assessment by patients and family caregivers and problems experienced by caregivers. Supportive Care in Cancer: Official Journal of the Multinational Association of Supportive Care in Cancer. 2015;**23**(7):1857-1864

[17] Armstrong P, Wilkinson P, McCorry NK. Use of parecoxib by continuous subcutaneous infusion for cancer pain in a hospice population. BMJ Supportive & Palliative Care. 2018;**8**(1):25-29

[18] Myers KG, Trotman IF. Use of ketorolac by continuous subcutaneous infusion for the control of cancer-related pain. Postgraduate Medical Journal. 1994;**70**(823):359-362

[19] Negro S, Martin A, Azuara ML, Sanchez Y, Barcia E. Stability of tramadol and haloperidol for continuous subcutaneous infusion at home. Journal of Pain and Symptom Management. 2005;**30**(2):192-199

[20] Mercadante S, Lodi F, Sapio M, Calligara M, Serretta R. Long-term ketamine subcutaneous continuous infusion in neuropathic cancer pain. Journal of Pain and Symptom Management. 1995;**10**(7):564-568

[21] Centeno C, Vara F. Intermittent subcutaneous methadone administration in the management of cancer pain. Journal of Pain & Palliative Care Pharmacotherapy. 2005;**19**(2):7-12

[22] Dickman A, Bickerstaff M, Jackson R, Schneider J, Mason S, Ellershaw J. Identification of drug combinations administered by continuous subcutaneous infusion that require analysis for compatibility and stability. BMC Palliative Care. 2017;**16**(1):22

[23] Campbell ML, Kiernan JM, Strandmark J, Yarandi HN. Trajectory of dyspnea and respiratory distress among patients in the last month of life. Journal of Palliative Medicine. 2018;**21**(2):194-199

[24] Guirimand F, Sahut d'izarn M, Laporte L, Francillard M, Richard JF, Aegerter P. Sequential occurrence of dyspnea at the end of life in palliative care, according to the underlying cancer. Cancer Medicine. 2015;**4**(4):532-539

[25] Okamoto Y, Morita T, Tsuneto S, Aoyama M, Kizawa Y, Shima Y, et al. Bereaved family members' perceptions of the distressing symptoms of terminal patients with cancer. American Journal of Hospice and Palliative Medicine. 2018;**35**(7):972-977

[26] Jansen K, Haugen DF, Pont L, Ruths S. Safety and effectiveness of palliative drug treatment in the last days of life-a systematic literature review. Journal of Pain and Symptom Management. 2018;**55**(2):508-21.e3

[27] Hadjiphilippou S, Odogwu SE, Dand P. Doctors' attitudes towards prescribing opioids for refractory dyspnoea: A single-centred study. BMJ Supportive & Palliative Care. 2014;**4**(2):190-192

[28] Puspawati N, Sitorus R, Herawati T. Hand-held fan airflow stimulation relieves dyspnea in lung cancer patients. Asia-Pacific Journal of Oncology Nursing. 2017;**4**(2):162-167

[29] Kako J, Morita T, Yamaguchi T, Kobayashi M, Sekimoto A, Kinoshita H, et al. Fan therapy is effective in relieving dyspnea in patients with terminally ill cancer: A parallel-arm, randomized controlled trial. Journal of Pain and Symptom Management. 2018;**56**(4):493-500

[30] Bennett MI. Death rattle: An audit of hyoscine (scopolamine) use and review of management. Journal of Pain and Symptom Management. 1996;**12**(4):229-233

[31] Lokker ME, van Zuylen L, van der Rijt CC, van der Heide A. Prevalence, impact, and treatment of death rattle: A systematic review. Journal of Pain and Symptom Management. 2014;**47**(1):105-122

[32] Likar R, Rupacher E, Kager H, Molnar M, Pipam W, Sittl R. Efficacy of glycopyrronium bromide and scopolamine hydrobromide in patients with death rattle: A randomized controlled study. Wiener Klinische Wochenschrift. 2008;**120**(21-22):679-683

[33] Wildiers H, Dhaenekint C, Demeulenaere P, Clement PM, Desmet M, Van Nuffelen R, et al. Atropine, hyoscine butylbromide, or scopolamine are equally effective for the treatment of death rattle in terminal care. Journal of Pain and Symptom Management. 2009;**38**(1):124-133

[34] Mercadante S, Marinangeli F, Masedu F, Valenti M, Russo D, Ursini L, et al. Hyoscine butylbromide for the management of death rattle: Sooner rather than later. Journal of Pain and Symptom Management. 2018;**56**(6):902-907

[35] Heisler M, Hamilton G, Abbott A, Chengalaram A, Koceja T, Gerkin R. Randomized double-blind trial of sublingual atropine vs. placebo for the management of death rattle. Journal of Pain and Symptom Management. 2013;**45**(1):14-22

[36] Shimizu Y, Miyashita M, Morita T, Sato K, Tsuneto S, Shima Y. Care strategy for death rattle in terminally ill cancer patients and their family members: Recommendations from a cross-sectional nationwide survey of bereaved family members' perceptions. Journal of Pain and Symptom Management. 2014;**48**(1):2-12

[37] Campbell ML, Yarandi HN. Death rattle is not associated with patient respiratory distress: Is pharmacologic treatment indicated? Journal of Palliative Medicine. 2013;**16**(10):1255-1259

[38] Lawlor PG, Gagnon B, Mancini IL, Pereira JL, Hanson J, Suarez-Almazor ME, et al. Occurrence, causes, and outcome of delirium in patients with advanced cancer: A prospective study. Archives of Internal Medicine. 2000;**160**(6):786-794

[39] Morita T, Akechi T, Ikenaga M, Inoue S, Kohara H, Matsubara T, et al. Terminal delirium: Recommendations from bereaved families' experiences. Journal of Pain and Symptom Management. 2007;**34**(6):579-589

[40] Bush SH, Lawlor PG, Ryan K, Centeno C, Lucchesi M, Kanji S, et al. Delirium in adult cancer patients: ESMO clinical practice guidelines. Annals of Oncology: Official Journal of the European Society for Medical Oncology (ESMO). 2018;**29**(Supplement_4):iv143-iiv65

[41] Agar MR, Lawlor PG, Quinn S, Draper B, Caplan GA, Rowett D, et al. Efficacy of oral risperidone, haloperidol, or placebo for symptoms of delirium among patients in palliative care: A randomized clinical trial. JAMA Internal Medicine. 2017;**177**(1):34-42

[42] Candy B, Jackson KC, Jones L, Leurent B, Tookman A, King M. Drug therapy for delirium in terminally ill adult patients. The Cochrane Database of Systematic Reviews. 2012;**11**:Cd004770

[43] Hui D, Frisbee-Hume S, Wilson A, Dibaj SS, Nguyen T, De La Cruz M, et al. Effect of lorazepam with haloperidol vs haloperidol alone on agitated delirium in patients with advanced cancer receiving palliative care: A randomized clinical trial. Journal of the American Medical Association. 2017;**318**(11):1047-1056

[44] Maltoni M, Scarpi E, Rosati M, Derni S, Fabbri L, Martini F, et al. Palliative sedation in end-of-life care and survival: A systematic review. Journal of Clinical Oncology: Official Journal of the American Society of Clinical Oncology. 2012;**30**(12):1378-1383

[45] Bruera S, Chisholm G, Dos Santos R, Crovador C, Bruera E, Hui D. Variations in vital signs in the last days of life in patients with advanced cancer. Journal of Pain and Symptom Management. 2014;**48**(4):510-517

[46] Hwang IC, Ahn HY, Park SM, Shim JY, Kim KK. Clinical changes in terminally ill cancer patients and death within 48 h: When should we refer patients to a separate room? Supportive Care in Cancer: Official Journal of the Multinational Association of Supportive Care in Cancer. 2013;**21**(3):835-840

[47] Hui D, Hess K, dos Santos R, Chisholm G, Bruera E. A diagnostic model for impending death in cancer patients: Preliminary report. Cancer. 2015;**121**(21):3914-3921

[48] Morita T, Ichiki T, Tsunoda J, Inoue S, Chihara S. A prospective study on the dying process in terminally ill cancer patients. American Journal of Hospice and Palliative Medicine. 1998;**15**(4):217-222

[49] Morita T, Tsunoda J, Inoue S, Chihara S. The palliative prognostic index: A scoring system for survival prediction of terminally ill cancer patients. Supportive Care in Cancer: Official Journal of the Multinational Association of Supportive Care in Cancer. 1999;**7**(3):128-133

[50] Glare PA, Eychmueller S, McMahon P. Diagnostic accuracy of the palliative prognostic score in hospitalized patients with advanced cancer. Journal of Clinical Oncology. 2004;**22**(23):4823-4828

[51] Gwilliam B, Keeley V, Todd C, Gittins M, Roberts C, Kelly L, et al. Development of prognosis in palliative care study (PiPS) predictor models to improve prognostication in advanced cancer: Prospective cohort study. British Medical Journal (Clinical Research Edition). 2011;**343**:d4920

[52] Uneno Y, Kanai M. Prognosis Prediction Models and their Clinical Utility in Palliative Care. In book: Highlights on Several Underestimated Topics in Palliative Care. Intech. 2017. DOI: 10.5772/intechopen.69663

[53] Hallenbeck J. Palliative care in the final days of life: "They were expecting it at any time". Journal of the American Medical Association. 2005;**293**(18):2265-2271

[54] Bailey FA, Williams BR. Preparation of residents for death pronouncement: A sensitive and supportive method. Palliative & Supportive Care. 2005;**3**(2):107-114

[55] Brown R, Dunn S, Byrnes K, Morris R, Heinrich P, Shaw J. Doctors' stress responses and poor communication performance in simulated bad-news consultations. Academic

Medicine: Journal of the Association of American Medical Colleges. 2009;**84**(11):1595-1602

[56] Schmidt TA, Norton RL, Tolle SW. Sudden death in the ED: Educating residents to compassionately inform families. The Journal of Emergency Medicine. 1992;**10**(5):643-647

[57] Sobczak K. The procedure for death notification-"In person, in time...". Anaesthesiology Intensive Therapy. 2013;**45**(4):241-243

[58] Marchand LR, Kushner KP, Siewert L. Death pronouncement: Survival tips for residents. American Family Physician. 1998;**58**(1):284-285

[59] Pollack M. Educating new resident physicians in death notification. Academic Medicine : Journal of the Association of American Medical Colleges. 1999;**74**(6):721

[60] Marchand L, Kushner K. Death pronouncements: Using the teachable moment in end-of-life care residency training. Journal of Palliative Medicine. 2004;**7**(1):80-84

[61] Hobgood C, Harward D, Newton K, Davis W. The educational intervention "GRIEV_ING" improves the death notification skills of residents. Academic Emergency Medicine. 2005;**12**(4):296-301

[62] Hobgood CD, Tamayo-Sarver JH, Hollar DW Jr, Sawning S. Griev_Ing: Death notification skills and applications for fourth-year medical students. Teaching and Learning in Medicine. 2009;**21**(3):207-219

[63] Nordstrom A, Fjellman-Wiklund A, Grysell T. Drama as a pedagogical tool for practicing death notification-experiences from Swedish medical students. BMC Medical Education. 2011;**11**:74

[64] Kusakabe A, Naito AS, Hirano K, Ikenaga K, Saitou N, Mikan H, et al. Death pronouncements: Recommendations based on a survey of bereaved family members. Journal of Palliative Medicine. 2016;**19**(6):646-651

[65] Hatano Y, Morita T, Otani H, Igarashi N, Shima Y, Miyashita M. Physician behavior toward death pronouncement in palliative care units. Journal of Palliative Medicine. 2018;**21**(3):368-372

[66] Ferrand E, Jabre P, Vincent-Genod C, Aubry R, Badet M, Badia P, et al. Circumstances of death in hospitalized patients and nurses' perceptions: French multicenter Mort-a-l'Hopital survey. Archives of Internal Medicine. 2008;**168**(8):867-875

Chapter 5

The Quality of Life of the Patients Under Palliative Care: The Features of Appropriate Assessment Tools and the Impact of Early Integration of Palliative Care

Thomas Antony Thaniyath

Abstract

Based on the WHO definition, the primary objective of palliative care (PC) is to improve the quality of life (QoL) of the patients facing life threatening illness by means of a multidisciplinary approach. The assessment of QoL in patients under PC is an important process for the identification of patient's overall conditions including psycho-social, spiritual issues as well as the evaluation of the services provided to the patient. The ideal assessment tool the measurement of QoL in patients under PC should be patient centered and contain both subjective and objective domains and be able to correlate with the definition of QoL. The factors which positively influence the extend of the QoL include, good doctor-patient communication, economic status, education, socio-economic support and spirituality. The negative factors are social isolation, lack of employment, poverty, rejection and stigmatization and experience of symptoms, such as uncontrolled pain. Early Integration of PC leads to higher psycho-social support and acceptance of diagnosis, and severity of illness, which in turn helps for the better symptom management and reduces the disease related stress, which clearly associated with improved QoL. It provides more time for the end of life decision making, promotes self-efficacy and sense of control in decision with respect to individual values.

Keywords: quality of life, palliative care, early palliative care, QoL assessment, QoL tools, symptom management, psycho-social support

1. Introduction

Palliative care is a philosophy based approach in patient care not on physical facilities but on attitudes and skills [1] and is redefined by the World Health Organization (WHO) in 2002 and extended to include palliative care for children for the active total care of patients facing life-threatening illness through prevention and relief of sufferings by means of early identification and impeccable assessment and treatment of pain and other problems as physical, psychosocial and spiritual, with an aim to improve the quality of life of the patient and their families [2, 3]. Most of the developed and developing countries recognized palliative medicine for the improvement

IntechOpen

of the quality of life of patients with chronic disease such as malignancy [4]. The primary goal of palliative care is the achievement of the best possible quality of life for the patients and their families and role extends to support on bereavement, if necessary. The term 'care' underpinned by the concept of total pain, defined as including not only physical symptoms but also mental distress and social or spiritual problems [5]. This concept of palliative care points to the need of holistic approach including symptom control for the management of the patients with terminal illness. Based on the above definition by WHO, the primary aim of palliative medicine is to prevent, treat the symptoms of patients with non-curable diseases as total care and to improve the quality of life (QoL) of the patient and their families.

The evaluation of QoL of patients in Palliative Care is an important procedure in the identification of a patient's overall condition as well as in the evaluation of the quality of service provided [6]. In patient's perspective, the following aspects such as physical abilities, personal autonomy, emotional state, socializing, spirituality, cognition, health care provision and preparation for death are important factors of quality of life in people with a life-limiting illness receiving palliative care [7] and to be considered during the assessment of quality of life in these patient cohort. The occurrence of incurable diseases can cause an enormous challenge to the patient, their family as well as medical professionals, affecting the QoL of patients in many ways [8]. With key components of systematic symptom assessment, pain control and other symptom relief, psychosocial support and family support, it is evident that early interdisciplinary palliative care and care givers' support help the patient to achieve effective symptom control and better quality in life [9]. However, usual practice to seek palliative care service is still limited to the terminal phase of illness. A coherent and empathetic communication of health professionals with the patient and their family has a major role in adopting patients' and their families' readiness for palliative care at the time of or shortly after diagnosis of incurable life-threatening illness [10–14]. In this context, this chapter highlights the facts with the primary objectives of:

1. To explain definitions and the variables for the terms "quality of life", and "Health Related Quality of Life (HRQoL)" in the concept of "Health"

2. To suggest appropriate research tools for the assessment of QoL and HRQoL in patients under palliative care

3. To describe the influence of palliative care medicine in the improvement of QoL in these patients.

2. Definitions and the variables for the assessment of QoL of patients under early palliative care

2.1 Definitions

Defining the QoL is challenging and many approaches based on human needs, subjective well-being, expectations and phenomenal viewpoints exists [15]. The available definitions of QoL that are useful in health care can be grouped into five categories:

1. Normal life

2. Happiness/satisfaction

3. Achievement of personal goals

4. Social utility and

5. Natural capacity [16].

As early as in 1949, Karnofsky outlined the necessity of assessment of patients' subjective improvement in terms of mood and attitude, general well-being and activity, appetite and alleviation of distressing symptoms such as pain, weakness and dyspnea in addition to performance status, length of remission and prolongation of life during the evaluation of new drugs in cancer chemotherapy and high lighlened the importance of psycho-social and QoL variables in molecule development. In contemporary terms, these subjective improvement criteria can be considered as QoL measurements and can be considered one of the first description on QoL in health care [17]. The alternative approach is with a view that individuals are the centre point to judge their own experiences and referred to as subjective QoL of subjective well-being (SWB) [18]. The subjective approach defines QoL as the congruence between aspirations and accomplishments, as perceived by the person and measures of life satisfaction, happiness, and positive and negative emotions falling in this category of subjective well-being [19]. These approaches direct to the necessity of a patient-centered approach for the evaluation of quality of life in the health care system. Since the introduction of the term "quality of life" in the medical literature in the 1960s, a number of researches have been happening, especially in patients with malignancy.

Based on a review, Aaronson [20] suggested two common threads in the structure and content of measures that carry the quality of life label.

1. Such measures tend to reflect a multidimensional conceptual approach. The following health dimensions are frequently incorporated to a greater or lesser degree in assessment of QoL.

   a. Physical health with variables such as somatic sensations, disease symptoms, and treatment related complications.

   b. Mental health ranging from a positive sense of well-being to non-pathological forms of psychological distress to diagnosable psychiatric disorders.

   c. Social health including qualitative and quantitative assessment of community contacts and interactions

   d. Functional health which includes both physical functioning in terms of self-care, mobility and physical activity as well as social role functioning in relation to family and work

Beyond these dimensions, other variables specific to a given disease may be incorporated, for example, quality of life evaluations in breast cancer will often include measures of sexual activities and body image. Another example studies in rheumatoid arthritis may include expanded assessment of joint mobility and pain.

2. The patient focused approach is primarily reliance on the subjective judgment of the patient themselves, rather than on observations of physicians, nurses, family members or other third parties. Although this process adds complexity to the data collection, considering the manner in which this approach

addresses the psychosocial factors surrounding disease and treatment, it is generally considered as the most appropriate.

This concept on QoL is supported by Ware [21] who suggested that routine assessment of a fairly broad, comprehensive set of psychosocial variables may often be most appropriate given our limited knowledge of the impact of chronic disease on everyday functioning, and of the psychosocial tradeoff associated with alternative treatments. Marcel [17] highlighted the importance of having a definition of QoL that covers the topic of research. Alternatively, he suggested getting umbrella coverage for any aspect of living with illness or disability to the term 'quality of life' in a QoL article. He advised the reader to focus on the variables which are actually measured in the study rather than the terms used.

In 1993, the WHO Quality of Life Group clarified the definition of the term Quality of Life as 'an individual's perception of their position in life in the context of the culture and value systems in which they live and in relation to their goals, expectations, standards and concerns. This broad concept on QoL is influenced by the individual's physical health, psychological state, level of independence, social relationships and their relationships to salient features of their environment in a complex manner [22]. However, at this point, it is important to consider the fact that the term QoL does not have same meaning to every person [23] and it is suggested that there are some aspects of QoL that are universal, where as some of them would be important only to the individual [24]. The interaction between these aspects-general and individual- will also vary from individual to individuals and their correlation is not static and moreover, changes overtime in response to life circumstances such as life-threatening or severity of illness [25]. Based on the above concepts and hypothesis, a number of definitions for QoL exist and many of them focus on subjective judgments. In view of this, a number of researchers have argued for the importance of inclusion of objective factors in the assessment of QoL [15]. Including all these variables in to consideration, QoL has been defined as "an overall general well-being which includes the objective assessments and subjective measurements of physical, material, social and emotional well-being together with the extent of personal development and purposeful activity, all weighted by a personal set of values" [26].

The term "Health- Related Quality of Life" appeared in published articles by the mid-1980s and it was defined as a subset of QoL, relating only to the health domain of that existence [15]. However, in 1994, Gill and Feinstein reviewed 75 articles titled with word quality of life and concluded that none of the article distinguished overall QoL from the HRQoL [27]. To reverse these situations, many theorists, researchers, organizations and the consensus groups have proposed definitions for QoL and HRQoL [17]. There are at least four definitions for HRQoL can be found in literature [15]. In 2010 Hays and Reeve defined HRQoL in terms of individual's functioning life and perception of well-being based on physical, mental and social domains of health [28]. Here functioning life represents the individual's ability to carry out some pre-defined activities, [28, 29] while wellbeing refers to an individual's subjective feelings [28].

In another article, Torrance WH, correlates QoL and HRQoL and quotes as "quality of life is an all-inclusive concept incorporating all factors that impact upon an individual's life. The Health Related QoL includes only those factors that are part of an individual's health". Non-health aspects of QoL are not included in HRQoL, for example economic and political factors [30]. Focusing on aspects of QoL affected by disease factors, in 1995 Ebrahim S provided a definition of HRQoL as "those aspects of self-perceived wellbeing that are related to or affected by the presence of disease or treatment" [31]. In another definition of HRQoL, Gold MR et al. focuses on the value of health and refer HRQoL to "the values assigned to different health states" [32].

2.2 Difference between the terms: Health, QoL and HRQoL

It is acknowledged that "health is only one dimension of quality of life" [16]. Satisfaction with life is influenced by health, but health status only explains a small part of life satisfaction outcomes [33]. Therefore we can consider the Health and QoL as distinct concepts [15]. As some of definitions of HRQoL indicate to health status of person and others resembles QoL, differentiation between HRQoL and both health status and QoL is more problematic [15]. Especially when considering, the first two definitions of HRQoL given above do not seem to add much to the concept of health. If HRQoL is considered as functioning and wellbeing in physical, psychological, and social domains, then we need to take HRQoL as a particular type of description of health, in view of the WHO definition of health. HRQoL describes health using functioning and well-being rather than, for example, in terms of clinical symptoms or biological variables [29]. It is thus should be considered as a type of health measure, but not a type of QoL measure. Similarly, if HRQoL is the health aspect of QoL then HRQoL should be considered as same as health condition. Particularly, the first two definitions of HRQoL, which included here do not distinguish HRQoL from that of health [15]. The third definition of HRQoL highlights the aspects of QoL that are indirectly influenced by health (e.g., health affects income and hence housing, education and so forth) [34]. Perhaps more reasonable is the variant of this definition, where HRQoL is the aspects of QoL most affected by ill health [15]. Qualitative research has observed that existence of a wide variety of non-health factors those are important to participants for evaluating their health states [35]. If the research participant's preferences are based on how health affects the QoL and if respondents estimate the effect of health status on QoL correctly then the utility of a health state could be referred to as health-related quality of life or more accurate term of 'health-adjusted quality of life' [15]. In summary, the above definitions of HRQoL reflect the values of definitions of both QoL and health in to its considerations.

2.3 The importance of HRQoL questionnaires measure in palliative care

As stated above, WHO defines palliative care as "an approach that improves the QoL of patients and their families facing the problems associated with life-threatening illness, through the prevention and relief of suffering by means of early identification and impeccable assessment and treatment of pain and other problems, physical, psychosocial, and spiritual" [36]. Since the patients under palliative care with chronic illness or non-curable disease, most of the measures in palliatives address for the symptom control and help the patients and their family to improve the quality of life physically, psycho-socially and spiritually. Based on the concept of above definition, the HRQoL questionnaire, such as the Personal Wellbeing Index (PWI) asks about satisfaction with: the standard of living, health, achievement, personal relationships, personal safety, community connectedness, and future security [37] in its assessment of variables. All these variables are more or less likely to be affected by ill health status of the individual. Because of this correlation between the domains and patient's perception on health status, it is recommendable that the QoL questionnaires could therefore be to measure self-perceived health status, unless the connection between measuring functioning and well-being and QoL is justified [15]. The domains of the two most validated assessment tools such as SF-6D and the EQ-5D would fit to the WHO health definition, although the questions range across the WHO classification scheme of impairment, activity limitation, and participation restriction. Yet, there have not been many explicit justifications for differentiating HRQoL from health status [15]. However, neither the EQ-5D nor the SF-6D contains patient valuation. Measures of HRQoL describe health status in terms of functioning health and wellbeing of individual than clinical parameters, and with a broad description of health condition than the measures of QoL. It is therefore more justified to classify typical HRQoL measures as measures of self-perceived health status [15]. So the ideal questionnaire should cover the concept of WHO definition along with patient self-evaluation on all aspect of QoL measures in relation his or her present health condition.

Spitzer et al. introduced a concise QL-index for measuring quality of life in cancer patients in 1981. This QoL instrument was based on the assessment of socio-personal variables and included physical, social, and emotional functions; attitude towards illness, personal features of patient's daily lives, including family interactions and the cost of illness. The considered items measures activities, self-care, general health, social support and out-look on life [38].

The findings in a systematic review by Nicola et al. [7] in 2016, with an objective to identify the aspects of QoL, which are important from the perspective of palliative care patients, suggests the following aspects as important for the quality of life in people with a life-limiting illness receiving palliative care on their own perspective: physical abilities, personal autonomy, emotional state, socializing, spirituality, cognition, health care provision and preparation for death. He also suggested a refinement of existing QoL measures in palliative care setting to improve the sensitivity and concluded with an opinion of generic preference based, HRQoL measures commonly used to inform public funding decisions do not include the domains such as cognition, emotional, physical, preparatory, social and the spirituality. Because of the existence of this mismatch between the domains available in assessment tools and the reality on the context of patient considerations, the assessment with the tools may fail to inform adequately on the money decisions about palliative care. Because of these mismatching facts, Carr and Higginson suggested for a patient-centered outcome measures (PCOMs), which capture the health status and well-being form the patient's perspective and focus on concern important to patient [24]. This point supported by Etkind et al., in a systematic review on the impact of PCOMs on processes and outcomes of palliative care, concluding that these type of measures raise the awareness of unmet need, improve recognition of symptoms and communication about QoL and benefit patient's emotional and psychological quality of life [39]. In short, during the selection of assessment tools for the evaluation of quality of life in patients under palliative care, it is recommendable for a patient centered outcome measuring questionnaire which correlate with definition of QoL.

3. The improvement of QOL of patients and their families under early palliative care

During early decades, palliative care services were initiated to provide a medical alternative to questionable medical practice regarding the end of life period: abandonment, euthanasia and inappropriate aggressive therapy and palliative care are usually offered late. Recently WHO recommends palliative care introduction as early as possible in the course of illness to increase the quality of life of patients and to positively influence the course of illness, in conjunction with other therapies, which are intended to prolong the life; such as chemotherapy or radiotherapy [40]. Palliative care is a multi-disciplinary approach that aims to improve the quality of life of all patients including both children and elderly and their families who are facing the challenges associated with life-threatening illness. These objectives of PC are achieved through the prevention and relief of sufferings, by means of early identification, assessment and treatment of pain and other physical, psychosocial and spiritual distress [40]. The WHO recommendations also support the use of necessary laboratory investigations for the better understanding and management of distressing clinical complications in these patient group.

3.1 The evidences supporting the early introduction of palliative care

The role of good doctor-patient communication is important in acceptance of illness, deciding the treatment options. With a focused intensified doctor-patient communication, early palliative care may lead to higher social support and increase the likelihood of the acceptance of the diagnosis and illness severity. This in turn improves the patient's openness to symptom control and psycho-social interventions, and thereby to reduce the disease related distress. The reduced distress itself associated with improved quality of life and consistently promotes survival [41–43]. Early palliative care intends to outline realistic and attainable goals of treatment and to facilitate patient's choices by providing adequate information and assessment of his or her values and preferences with regard to advance care planning [44, 45]. In a systematic review of a small number of trials, Haun MW et al. found that early palliative care interventions may have more beneficial effects on quality of life and symptom intensity among patients with advanced cancer than among those given usual/standard cancer care alone. Apart from small effect size of the studies, they observed the findings may be clinically relevant at an advanced disease stage with limited prognosis, at which time further decline in quality of life is very common [46].

There are evidences that under early palliative care patient and family members are better informed on disease symptoms and severity and treatment directives and are provided with more time for end of life decisions, which promotes the experience of higher self-efficacy and sense of control in decisions with respect to the individual values [47]. It is proved that, the effective use of palliative care in linked with less aggressive cancer treatment, such as reduced use of questionable chemotherapeutic agents and treatments and this practice will de-escalate treatment intensity in final, irreversible health conditions [48]. The above observations is also supported by Temel et al. in 2010 [49] with their findings in a randomized trial with participation of 151 patients of newly diagnosed metastatic non-small cell carcinoma. The primary objective of this study was improvement in quality of life and overall survival as secondary objective. In their study, it has been observed that the patients in group of early palliative care service along with standard oncologic treatment showed significant improvement in quality of life and in mood, than the patients in the group of standard oncology treatment only. In addition, the patients with early palliative care led a significantly longer survival (p = 0.02), despite less aggressive end of life care. In view of the observations in this randomized controlled trail, American Society of Clinical Oncology supported the combined use standard oncology treatment along with palliative care in the course of illness for any patients with metastatic cancer.

The early integration of palliative care service for the treatment of cancer patients especially with metastasis is also supported by, Pirl et al. [50] in 2012, with the observations in their trial. It claimed that early introduction of palliative care improved the result of medical comorbidity management, including depression and helps in the discontinuation of inappropriate and possibly detrimental cancer treatment at the end of life. Recently, Hutt et al. [51] conducted a phase III randomized trial in 2018, with an aim to test the hypothesis that the use of early palliative care provides greater clinical benefits than standard practice for a population of patients with metastatic upper gastro-intestinal cancers. The primary objective in this study was overall survival. The authors concluded with expectation of integration of earlier palliative care in oncologic care of patients with metastatic gastro-intestinal cancer.

3.2 The factors should be addressed under palliative care for the betterment of quality of life in patients

In 2011 Jacoba et al. [25] studied the effect of palliative care in a resource poor community in South Africa, with the themes of:

a. the factors that had a positive influence on quality of life,

b. factors that had a negative influence on quality of life

c. experience of quality of life.

In their study, it is observed that: being able to work as a very important factor for all the participants involved in the study, as it keeping them busy and having no time to spend for unnecessary worries in addition to help in earnings. Support from friends and family as well as health care professionals was another major factor contributing for the improvement of quality of life. Spiritual activities such as going to church, participating church services, singing in choir and prayers made the participants to feel strong and comfort and gave them a feel of "alright". Lastly, comes the symptom control. The poverty was the predominant negative factor on the quality of life of the study participants. Other negative factors were unemployment, separation from children, rejection and stigmatization and experiencing the symptoms with pain as mostly described symptom. It is observed that uplifting of education and economic status of the community will help for the improved psycho-social support extending to the terminally ill patients and there by their quality of life [52].

4. Conclusion

The primary objective of palliative care is to improve the QoL of the patients facing life threatening illness by means of a multidisciplinary approach. The process of QoL assessment identifies the patient's overall conditions including psycho-social, spiritual issues as well as the evaluation of the services provided to him. So the ideal assessment tool the measurement of QoL in patients under palliative care should be patient centered and contain both subjective and objective domains and be able to correlate with the definition of QoL. It is evident that early integration of palliative care improves the QoL of patients with terminally ill condition and Early adaptation of palliative care is advisable for the management of patients with chronic conditions such as cancer.

Conflict of interest

None.

Author details

Thomas Antony Thaniyath
Faculty of Medicine, University of Tabuk, Tabuk, Saudi Arabia

*Address all correspondence to: thaniyan1@gmail.com

References

[1] Saunders C. The evolution of palliative care. Journal of the Royal Society of Medicine. 2001;**94**:430-432

[2] World Health Organization. Cancer Pain Relief and Palliative Care. Geneva: WHO; 2002

[3] WHO. Definition of Palliative Care. Available from: www.who.int/cancer/palliative/definition/en

[4] Manual of Cancer Services Standard. London: National Health Services; 2000

[5] Saunders C. The symptomatic treatment of incurable malignant disease. Prescribers Journal. 1964;**4**:68-73

[6] Correia FR, Carlo MMPRD. Evaluation of quality of life in a palliative care context: An integrative literature review. Revista Latino-Americana de Enfermagem. 2012;**20**(2):401-410. www.eerp.usp.br/rlae

[7] Nicola MC, Bradley S, Julie R, David CC. What aspects of quality of life are important from palliative care patients' perspective? A systematic review of qualitative research. Journal of Pain and Symptom Management. 2016;**52**(2):318-328. DOI: 10.1016/jpainsymman.2016.02.012

[8] Addington HJ, McCarthy M. Dying from cancer: Results of a national population based investigation. Palliative Medicine. 1995;**9**:295-305

[9] Hui D, De La Cruz M, Mori M, Parsons HA, Kwon JH, Torres-Vigil, et al. Concepts and definitions of 'supportive care', 'best supportive care', "palliative care" and "hospice care" in the published literature, dictionaries, and text books. Supportive Care in Cancer. 2013;**21**:659-685. DOI: 10.1007/s00520-012-1564-y

[10] de Haes H, Teunissen S. Communication in palliative care: A review of recent literature. Current Opinion in Oncology. 2005;**17**:345-350

[11] Dowsett SM, Saul JL, Butow PN, Dunn SM, Boyer MJ, Findlow R, et al. Communication styles in the cancer consultation: Preferences for a patient-centred approach. Psycho-Oncology. 2000;**9**:147-156

[12] Meyers FJ, Linder J. Simultaneous care: Disease treatment and palliative care throughout illness. Journal of Clinical Oncology. 2003;**21**:1412-1415

[13] Morrison RS, Meier DE. Clinical practice. Palliative care. New England Journal of Medicine. 2004;**350**:2582-2590

[14] Sinclair CT. Communicating a prognosis in advanced cancer. Journal of Supportive Oncology. 2006;**4**:201-204

[15] Milad K, John B. Health, health-related quality of life, and quality of life: What is the difference? PharmacoEconomics. 2016;**34**(7):645-649

[16] Ferrans CE. Quality of life: Conceptual issues. Seminars in Oncology Nursing. 1990;**6**:248-254

[17] Marcel VM. Definitions of quality of life: What has happened and how to move on. Topics in Spinal Cord Injury Rehabilitation. 2014;**20**(3):167-180

[18] Fuhrer MJ. Subjectifying quality of life as medical rehabilitation outcome. Disability and Rehabilitation. 2000;**22**:481-489

[19] Dijkers M. Quality of life after spinal cord injury: A meta-analysis of the effects of disablement components. Spinal Cord. 1997;**35**(12):829-840

[20] Aaronson NK. Quantitative issues in health-related quality of life assessment. Health Policy. 1988;**10**(3):217-230

[21] Ware JE Jr. Conceptualizing disease impact and treatment outcomes. Cancer. 1984;**53**:2217-2384

[22] Bowling A. Health Related Quality of Life: A Discussion of the Concept, Its Use and Measurement Background: 'The Quality of Life'. Available from: http://info.worldbank.org/etools/docs/library/48475.m2s5bowling.pdf

[23] Chippendale S. Choice at the end of life: Ethics and palliative care. In: Kinghorn S, Gaines S, editors. Palliative Nursing: Improving End of Life Care. 2nd ed. Bailierre Tindal, Elsevier; 2002. pp. 171-190

[24] Carr AJ, Higginson IJ. Are quality of life measures patient centered? BMJ. 2001;**322**:1357-1360

[25] Jacoba JJVR, Johanna EM, Corrien VB. Quality oflife from the perspective of the palliative care patient in a resource-poor community in South Africa. Palliative & Supportive Care. 2013;**11**:21-28. DOI: 10.1017/S1478951512000430

[26] Felce D, Perry J. Quality of life: Its definition and measurement. Research in Developmental Disabilities. 1995;**16**:51-74

[27] Gill TM, Feinstein AR. A critical appraisal of the quality of quality of life measurements. JAMA. 1994;**271**(8):619-626

[28] Hays RD, Reeve BB. Measurement and modeling of health-related quality of life. In: Killewo J, Heggenhougen HK, Quah SR, editors. Epidemiology and Demography in Public Health. San Diego: Academic Press; 2010. pp. 195-205

[29] Wilson IB, Cleary PD. Linking clinical variables with health-related quality of life. A conceptual model of patient outcomes. JAMA. 1995;**273**:59-65

[30] Torrance GW. Utility approach to measuring health-related quality of life. Journal of Chronic Diseases. 1987;**40**(6):593-600

[31] Ebrahim S. Clinical and public health perspectives and applications of health-related quality of life measurement. Social Science & Medicine. 1995;**41**:1383-1394

[32] Gold MR, Patrick DL, Torrance GW, Fryback D, Hadorn DC, Kamlet M, et al. Identifying and valuing outcomes. In: Gold MR, Siegel JE, Russell LB, Weinstein MC, editors. Cost-Effectiveness in Health and Medicine. Oxford: Oxford University Press; 1996

[33] Michalos A. Social indicators research and health-related quality of life research. Social Indicators Research. 2004;**65**:27-72

[34] Leplège A, Hunt S. The problem of quality of life in medicine. Journal of the American Medical Association. 1997;**278**:47-50

[35] Baker R, Robinson A. Responses to standard gambles: Are preferences "well-constructed"? Health Economics. 2004;**13**:37-48

[36] Yun YH, Kang EK, Lee J, et al. Development and validation of the quality care questionnaire-palliative care (QCQ-PC): Patient-reported assessment of quality of palliative care. BMC Palliative Care. 2018;**17**(1):40. DOI: 10.1186/s12904-018-0296-2

[37] Lau ALD, Cummins RA, McPherson W. An investigation into the cross-cultural equivalence of the Personal Wellbeing Index. Social Indicators Research. 2005;**72**:403-430

[38] Spitzer WO, Dobson AJ, Hall J, et al. Measuring the quality of life of cancer

patients. A concise QL-index for use by physicians. Journal of Chronic Diseases. 1981;**34**:584-597

[39] Etkind SN, Daveson BA, Kwok W, et al. Capture, transfer and feedback of patient-centered outcomes data in palliative care populations: Does it make difference? A systematic review. Journal of Pain and Symptom Management. 2015;**49**:611-624

[40] http://www.who.int/ncds/management/palliative-care/en/ [Accessed: November 29, 2018]

[41] Gotay CC, Kawamoto BA, Efficace F. The prognostic significance of patient-reported outcomes in cancer clinical trials. Journal of Clinical Oncology. 2008;**26**:1355-1368. DOI: 10.1200/JCO.2007.13.3439

[42] Irwin KE, Greer JA, Khatib J, Temel JS, Pirl WF. Early palliative care and metastatic non-small cell lung cancer: Potential mechanism of prolonged survival. Chronic Respiratory Disease. 2012;**10**:35-47. DOI: 10.1177/1479972312471549

[43] Pinquart M, Dubersstein PR. Depression and cancer mortality: A meta-analysis. Psychological Medicine. 2010;**40**:1797-1810. DOI: 10.1017/s0033291709992285

[44] Levy MH, Adolph MD, Back A, Block S, Codada SN, Dalal S, et al. Palliative care. Journal of the National Comprehensive Cancer Network. 2012;**10**:1284-1309

[45] Van Mechelen W, Aertgeerts B, De Ceulaer K, Thoonsen B, Vermandere M, Warmenhoven F, et al. Defining palliative care patient: A systematic review. Palliative Medicine. 2013;**27**: 197-208. DOI: 10.1177/0269216311435268

[46] Haun MW, Estel S, Rücker G, Friederich HC, Villalobos M, Thomas M, et al. Early palliative care for adults with advanced cancer. Cochrane Database of Systematic Reviews. 2017;**6**:CD011129. DOI: 10.1002/14651858.CD011129.pub2

[47] CS MC, Rosenfeld B, Breitbart W. Effect of spiritual well-being on end of life despair in terminally ill cancer patients. Lancet. 2003;**361**:1603-1607. DOI: 10.1177/0269216311435268

[48] Earle CC, Landrum MB, Souza JM, Neville BA, Weeks JC, Ayanian JZ. Aggressiveness of cancer care near the end of life: Is it a quality of care issue? Journal of Clinical Oncology. 2008;**26**:3860-3866. DOI: 10.1200/JCO.2007.15.8253

[49] Temel JS, Greer JA, Muzikansky A, et al. Early palliative care for patients with metastatic non-small cell lung cancer. The New England Journal of Medicine. 2010;**363**:733-742

[50] Pirl WF, Greer JA, Traeger L, et al. Depression and survival in metastatic non-small cell lung cancer: Effects of early palliative care. Journal of Clinical Oncology. 2012;**30**:1310-1315

[51] Hutt E, Da Silva A, Bogart E, Sara Le LD, Pannier D, Stephane D, et al. Impact of early palliative care on overall survival of patients with metastatic upper gastrointestinal cancers treated with first-line chemotherapy: A randomised phase III trial. BMJ Open. 2018;**88**:e015904. DOI: 10.1136/bmjopen-2017-015904

[52] Antony T, Merghani TH. The influence of demographic factors on social affections among chronic patients under home based nursing care. AARJSH. 2015;**2**(7):166-175

Chapter 6

Palliative Care Network in Brazil

Juliana Guimarães Lima Munis, Juliana Dias Reis Pessalacia, Jacqueline Resende Boaventura, Ana Paula Da Silva, Luciana Ferreira Da Silva, Aires Garcia dos Santos Júnior and Adriano Menis Ferreira

Abstract

Brazil is a country with great diversity and distinct realities, so there is a proportional challenge and complexity in offering a unified and integrated system which is accessible, of quality, and effective. Population aging and the increased incidence of chronic-degenerative noncommunicable diseases (NCDs) increase the need for palliative care (PC); however, public policies still need to be implemented so that this care encompasses adequate funding, professional training, and guaranteed medication. The first national policy for PC was recently proposed, providing guidelines for the organization of PC, emphasizing the importance of integration between the different levels of care and services in the Brazilian health system (SUS). Nevertheless, the challenges of this policy include the training of professionals, communication in the network, the absence of integrated health information systems, and effective mechanisms to finance this new modality of care.

Keywords: palliative care, health services, primary healthcare, health policy, community integration

1. Introduction

Populations have specific health preferences and needs, with characteristics manifested in demographic and epidemiological analyses. Health systems are organized according to each demand of this process [1].

Demographic data show that Brazilian population, mostly composed of young people, is changing. Life expectancy is simultaneously growing with the number of elderly people, while the number of births is decreasing [2].

Population aging results in a greater demand for health services and palliative care (PC). Chronic conditions, strongly related to this process, require special attention, and the reorganization of the system aimed at health promotion and healthy living habits is part of this new reality [3].

Currently, the Brazilian care model is fragmented, and there is an imbalance between preventive and curative actions, with predominance of medical care and focus on acute conditions [4].

The challenge and the complexity of providing a unified and integrated system which is accessible, of quality, and effective are proportional to the size of a country with great diversities and distinct realities [5].

All this complexity includes social plurality, more than one level of multidisciplinary and multiprofessional care, which receives resources from various sources and presents structural and technological inequality [4].

The organization of health has isolated levels that do not communicate with each other. Primary healthcare (PHC) is not related to secondary care, and none of them are related to tertiary care [1]. Thus, the lack of communication between healthcare levels prevents comprehensive care [6].

Comprehensiveness is part of the guidelines of the Unified Health System (SUS). It is a guiding concept of care that aims at treating each individual with respect, in his/her totality, valuing his/her needs and characteristics [7].

The healthcare networks (HCN) emerge within this context, mainly to interconnect the care levels and to integrate care itself [4].

The concept of HCN proposes a polyarchy, i.e., democratic, person-centered structure where health services communicate at all levels, and no level is more or less important than the other. It allows comprehensive care with promotional, preventive, curative, caregiving, rehabilitative, and palliative interventions. Thus, it offers a humanized and quality service to the population [8].

The Administrative Rule 4279, of December 30, 2010, regulates HCNs. It establishes guidelines for the organization of HCNs within the scope of the SUS. The networking system was necessary for a better health policy, a new structure based on the covenants for health, life, and in defense of the SUS, which assume responsibility for the regionalization and the health situation of Brazil and for strengthening the policy, principles, and guidelines of the SUS. PHC is the major coordinator of care, the gateway and communication center between users and health professionals. It distributes and redistributes assistance for all levels of healthcare horizontally, according to the needs. This explains the concept of networks [5].

The basic elements for the development of networks are well-defined population, based on registers performed on primary care level; operational structure, i.e., the relationship between the three different care levels of the network; care models, which are characterized in acute conditions that need technologies and also depend on the physiological response of each individual/community; and models of chronic conditions, in which promotion, prevention, rehabilitation, and palliative care actions take place [9].

Structurally, the heath network presents the following aspects: management to articulate PHC activities with the other levels, support systems, pharmaceutical assistance, health information systems, logistic systems, user identification, clinical records, systems of regulated access to care, and transport systems, as well as a communication center that coordinates flow and counterflow in the care system [3].

The network system is quite innovative when compared to the fragmented one currently disseminated; however, obstacles are expected in new deployments, both due to the simple fact of the change and due to old unresolved problems in health. It is necessary to know the needs of the population to establish a fluid and organized flow of work. This adaptation allows healthcare levels not to be isolated and provides for the movement of people through the network. However, the reality is somewhat different, as the operation is complex, bureaucratic, and disjointed, often compromising the speed of service and its potential for problem-solving [4].

The care level that is closest to people's lives is the primary care, playing a vital role within the system. On the other hand, primary care has not been adequately qualified. Moreover, the difficulty to access the secondary level, specialized consultations, and diagnostic and therapeutic support services also demonstrates the fragility of the HCN [6].

Structural and bureaucratic issues are factors that hinder the comprehensiveness of care, as well as the passivity in the actions of the PHC [9].

DOI: http://dx.doi.org/10.5772/intechopen.85169

Health professionals, as the key elements of the care system, experience all these complex obstacles in daily basis. They do not recognize the role they play within the network and are still attached to bureaucratic and inflexible routines [4].

Another study on the knowledge of professionals about this subject points out their lack of information regarding the healthcare levels available and their articulation [9].

Currently, the aforementioned population aging and the increased incidence in chronic-degenerative noncommunicable diseases have increased the need for palliative care. However, it is still necessary to implement public policies for the adequate financing of care, training of professionals, and provision of medications [10].

This chapter aims to present the political perspectives for the organization of a HCN for palliative care in Brazil.

2. Political perspectives of palliative care in the healthcare network

The term "palliative" comes from the Latin term *pallium*, whose definition is "blanket," "cover." It was used to describe the robes offered to the pilgrims when they left the hospices. The purpose of this clothing was protecting them from the weather during the trips. At present, the word "palliative," besides encompassing the notion of embracement and protection, contemplates the valuation of care to the human being based on a holistic approach [11].

Population aging causes the expansion of chronic-degenerative and incapacitating diseases, a fact that interferes in public health and in the capacity of provision of care by families and institutions [12].

Thus, PC in the twenty-first century basically consists in a skill that health professionals develop to care for the suffering of patients and their families facing life-threatening health situations [13].

Statistics released in 2012 by the Worldwide Palliative Care Alliance indicate that about 18 million people died on the planet suffering irrelevant pain due to inappropriate access to pain treatment. In Brazil, PC was introduced in the 1980s, and palliative medicine became a recognized medical area in 2011. Quality of life and symptom relief are crucial in this context [14].

However, in Brazil, the practice of PC has been evolving since the late 1990s. Official information from the National Academy of Palliative Care (NAPC) published in 2006 pointed out about 40 influential teams and 300 hospital beds assigned for such care [15].

Although primary care is the lowest cost strategy and has full impact on public health, the provision of PC in Brazil is still hospital-centered [13].

In view of this deficiency of care measures in primary care, it is necessary to raise the population's awareness. However, this awareness will only happen through the expansion of knowledge about PC, clarifying the history, implementation, functionality, and applicability of PC.

The origin of the philosophy of PC is linked to the emergence of hospices (guesthouses). Hospices originated in the Middle Ages, and their outbreak influenced the pilgrimages of Christians to the holy places, due to the long distances traveled for months and even years [16].

The first hospice that demonstrated a holistic view of the human person was the St. Christopher's Hospice, in London. It was created in the 1960s, in the twentieth century, by a nurse, physician, and social worker called Cicely Saunders. Saunders's concern was to provide humanized care through pain relief and symptom control [16].

In 1990, the World Health Organization (WHO) established a definition for PC, which encompasses care measures and treatments aimed at pain relief in order to promote a better quality of life for terminally ill patients and their families. However, this definition initially applied only to cancer patients [15].

The Oncology Therapeutic Support Center was inaugurated in 1998. This was a hospital sector exclusively dedicated to PC. This is the first of a series of internal restructuring actions in the institute with the purpose of making the practice of cancerology more focused on the weighted provision of services to the population [17].

Thus, historically, the concept of PC was initially linked to cancer patients [18], but it was subsequently extended, although insufficiently, for patients in later stages of other chronic diseases that had similar needs [19, 20].

The history of PC is relatively contemporary in Brazil, the course of this discussion contributed to health professionals' understanding about the philosophy given to patients without prognosis of cure, thus promoting the process of care and valuation of the human being [21].

In order to implement palliative care for patients with pain, the Ministry of Health established the National Program for Pain Relief and Palliative Care within the SUS in 2002, through the Administrative Rule MS/GM no. 198 [10].

The Administrative Rule MS/GM no. 198 was revoked by the Administrative Rule MS/GM no. 3.150/2006, which established the Technical Council for Pain Control and Palliative Care, and this council began to be responsible for national guidelines on pain control and PC, for the organization of care networks in this context, and for training and qualifying professionals to address pain control. Policies directed to PC are of paramount importance for a quality care, ruled under the law [10].

The Brazilian Council of Medicine (CFM, in Portuguese), the body that regulates and supervises medical practice, has published different resolutions directly related to this topic and that will certainly promote important reflections and advances in this area. Four of these resolutions are worth mentioning, namely, resolution on the legitimacy of orthothanasia (CFM Resolution 1.805/06); resolution on the new Code of Medical Ethics, where PC is directly mentioned (CFM Resolution 1931/09); rule that defines palliative medicine as an area of action (CFM Resolution 1973/12); and CFM Resolution 1995/12, on advance directives [15].

The lack of a public policy on PC in Brazil is no longer a fateful reality because a resolution was approved (Resolution no. 41, October 31, 2018) with guidelines for the organization of PC in the light of continued care in the SUS, the Tripartite Interagency Committee, in the use of the attributions granted by item II of Art. 14-A of Law no. 8080, of September 19, 1990, and the provisions of item I of Art. 32 of Decree 7.508, of June 28, 2011, in accordance with item II of the sole paragraph of Art. 87 of the Brazilian Constitution [22, 23].

It is estimated that PC is needed in about 40–60% of all deaths worldwide. However, in 2014, it was estimated that only 14% of the patients who needed these care received it, and 78% of these people lived in low- and middle-income countries [24].

According to the Worldwide Palliative Care Alliance, even if more than 100 million people would benefit annually from PC (including family members and caregivers), less than 8% of those who need this type of care would have their access guaranteed. In our reality, training in PC is rarely included in the educational curriculum of health professionals. In addition, the availability of pain drugs—the most basic topic when it comes to minimizing patient suffering—is woefully inadequate in most parts of the world, often because of concerns about its illicit use and drug trafficking [15].

In Brazil, it is estimated that between 521,000 and 536,000 people need PC, but this type of care tends to be indicated only in the end-of-life phase, restricting the performance of specialized teams in this area [25]. The WHO proposes the early initiation of PC and that this care walks together to curative treatment, seeking a better understanding of the actions, control of symptoms, and quality of life of the patients [26].

Providing PC since the beginning of the curative treatment makes it possible for the patients and their families to contact with the health team. As the chronic progressive disease evolves and the curative treatment loses effectiveness in controlling or modifying it, PC becomes more necessary and even exclusive because of the scenario of incurability. This management ensures the construction of a bond of trust between the patient-family-team triad, facilitating and contributing to the articulation and development of strategic plans of comprehensive and continuous assistance [27].

The *Economist* magazine evaluated the quality of death in 80 countries through the possibility of access to opioids, the existence of public policies focused on PC, and access to PC in health services. Brazil ranked 42nd, behind Chile, Costa Rica, Panama, Argentina, Uruguay, South Africa, Uganda, Mongolia, or Malaysia. Thus, in Brazil, many patients with severe diseases experience uncontrolled pain and do not receive palliative care [13].

PC is complex care dealing with physical, psychosocial, and spiritual problems at the end of life [28]. When faced with a life-threatening illness, most would rather die at home [29].

Available data indicate that most people around the world prefer to spend the last phase of their lives at home. To respect this preference and avoid or minimize overcrowding in hospitals, PC is necessary in PHC and home care. PHC physicians with basic PC training, availability of correct medications, and simple, safe, effective, and inexpensive equipment can effectively respond to the needs of these patients during home-based PC. The implementation of PC integrated into PHC can be of high quality and low cost for health systems and reduce dependence on outpatient and inpatient hospital services [24].

Given this context, the Brazilian SUS has perceived the need to improve health services to meet the PC and, therefore, has encouraged further studies that seek to broaden the qualification of healthcare professionals and to ensure continued care. Despite these efforts, the offer of PC is still hospital-centered, and yet only 10% of these institutions have a specific team for PC [13].

The inclusion of PC in PHC implies the execution of actions planned for this level of care and the coordination of care to users, respecting the WHO's precepts and guaranteeing comprehensiveness through the organization of HCNs. In this perspective, PHC is the best level of care for the provision and coordination of PC, since it has the potential to develop actions that favor quality of life and continuity of care, both inside and outside the home. Furthermore, care is provided close to the patient's families, avoiding unnecessary hospitalizations and decreasing the risk for infections [30].

Patients eligible for PC may need care with distinct complexities, which requires integration between the levels of care. Thus, early identification of patients eligible for PC has benefits, as aggressive diagnostic and therapeutic interventions are avoided, and unnecessary suffering and costs are reduced [31, 32].

Therefore, it is necessary to articulate the different components of the health system, creating a mechanism of reference and counter-reference for cases of clinical intercurrence [25].

According to the WHO [24], the implementation of a home-based PC service involves eight necessary steps:

1. Evaluation of patient needs and available resources

2. Establishment of formalization of the organization through reference terms and registration with authorities

3. Creation of a plan of action (which resources will be needed, how they can be obtained, target audience and services that will be covered)

4. Recruitment and development of an ongoing training program

5. Mobilization of resources

6. Integration within the health system, associating PC with the primary and tertiary care of the operator

7. Dissemination of the service

8. Encouragement of the participation of associations, groups, and students

In Brazil, PHC was implemented in 2006 through the Family Health Strategy, based on the ordinance of the Cabinet of the Minister/Ministry of Health No. 648, of March 28, 2006. Through this ordinance, home-based care becomes one of the tasks of PHC teams, especially FHS teams, which since their regulation have among their attributions the realization of care actions in the basic health unit, at the home of patients, and in the community [33].

However, on May 27, 2013, the Administrative Rule CM/MS no. 963 redefined home-based care within the scope of the SUS by reorganizing the work process of teams that provide home-based care in primary, outpatient, emergency, and hospital services, with a view to reducing the demand for hospital care and/or the length of hospitalization, promoting humanization of care, deinstitutionalization, and increase of autonomy of users [34].

This ordinance also presents the role of PHC in home-based PC, assigned as home-based care type 1 (HC1), with the goal of serving the population with the following characteristics: patients who have health problems controlled/compensated and with physical difficulty or impossibility of reaching a health unit and those requiring less complex care, with less frequency, and with less need for health resources [35].

This level of care (HC1) is integrated into two levels of home-based care (HC2 and HC3) carried out by home-based care multiprofessional teams (HCMT) intended for this purpose, upon the need of integration between levels. The role of the HCMT does not replace actions carried out at homes by PHC teams, especially the Family Health Strategy teams. On the contrary, by considering HC1 as the responsibility of these teams, the Ministry of Health recognizes that their work is a crucial axis, while the HCMT presents themselves as a complementary possibility, when the demands of the patients go beyond the solving capacity of PHC teams [33].

However, it is difficult to include PC in the context of PHC due to the lack of understanding of the professionals involved in this care and the difficulty of establishing an open and honest communication with the family. Moreover, providing training on PC seems not to be a priority for managers. In this line, there is a lack of subjects on the training of health professionals addressing this theme in the curricula, reinforcing that experience in PC comes with practice [30].

Therefore, the approach of PC in the HC area and also the recognition of HC as a space of great importance for the implementation of PC are pertinent.

The humanistic principles that guide PC are in line with those that guide HC, but the applicability of these principles in the context of HC in the public health system in Brazil is insufficient, valuing the curativist, technicist, and biologic aspects of care [36].

In view of all the political context involving health in Brazil and based on the experiences of other countries in the elaboration and implementation of specific policies aimed at patients eligible for PC, through Resolution No. 41 of October 31, 2018, the Ministry of Health provided the guidelines for the organization of PC in the light of continuous integrated care within the SUS [24]:

Article 5 PC shall be offered at any point in the healthcare network, namely:

I. Primary care: it is the network coordinator and care coordinator and will be responsible for following up users with life-threatening illnesses in its territory, with predominance of longitudinal care provided by primary care teams along with the expanded Family Health Center (NASF), with the support of the rest of the care network, whenever necessary.

II. Home-based care: the home-based care teams, whose modality will be defined based on the intensity of care, observing the unique therapeutic plan, should contribute to preparing the patient's home to be the main *locus* of care in the end of life, whenever possible. It will be indicated for people who need PC in bedridden situation or restricted to home, whenever this is considered the most appropriate care offer.

III. Ambulatory care: it should be structured to meet the PC demands from other levels of care of the network.

IV. Emergency care: the services will provide care to relieve acute symptoms, focused on the comfort and dignity of the person, according to the best practices and available evidence.

V. Hospital care: focused on the control of symptoms that cannot be controlled at another level of care.

In addition to the resolution presented by the Ministry of Health, there are other concerns, such as the elaboration of guidelines that guarantee the comprehensiveness and continuity of PC at all levels of care within the HCN with appropriate communication and commitment of the parties involved. It is necessary to establish means of accreditation for other services that need to integrate the network in a complementary manner because, according to studies, the growth of PC units or groups throughout Brazil is still very incipient. Providing technical and higher levels of training for teams is also an important item for consolidating the humanization of this care and raising awareness among professionals [37]. Studying the experiences of other countries is essential for the elaboration of proposals and optimization of resources.

Another important aspect to be mentioned is the need to broaden the articulation between the various health information systems with a view to subsidizing the evaluation of actions developed and decision-making. The broadening of communication between health systems favors the improvement of the quality of services and of management [38].

Prior to the implementation of the National Palliative Care Policy, isolated actions were carried out through initiatives of sectors within the health services concerned with the implementation of strategies for pain relief, which clearly shows the scarcity of resources invested in PC. The implementation of PC is a challenge that requires commitment and investment from the government [39].

Therefore, the publication of this resolution is only the beginning of the path for regulation of PC in Brazil. New objectives need to be drawn so that the implementation of PC becomes effective and adequate to the Brazilian reality, providing comprehensiveness to the assistance and PC in its essence.

3. Conclusion

Brazil has public policies focused on HCN in different types of assistance, with PHC as the driver of the network. However, the discussion about the organization of PC is still recent and demands major challenges. The first national policy for PC was recently proposed in the country, providing guidelines for the organization of PC and highlighting the importance of integration between the different levels of care and services in SUS. However, there are challenges for this policy, such as the training of professionals, communication within the network, and the lack of integrated health information systems and of effective mechanisms for financing this new modality of care in the country.

Acknowledgements

We thank the Foundation for Research Support of Mato Grosso do Sul (FUNDECT) and the Ministry of Health (PPSUS) for the financial support to the study that is linked to this work.

Conflict of interests

We declare that there is no conflict of interests in the accomplishment of this research.

Author details

Juliana Guimarães Lima Munis, Juliana Dias Reis Pessalacia*,
Jacqueline Resende Boaventura, Ana Paula Da Silva, Luciana Ferreira Da Silva,
Aires Garcia dos Santos Júnior and Adriano Menis Ferreira
Federal University of Mato Grosso do Sul, Três Lagoas, Mato Grosso do Sul, Brazil

*Address all correspondence to: juliana@pessalacia.com.br

References

[1] Mendes EV. As Redes de Atenção à Saúde. Organização Pan-Americana da Saúde: Brasília, DF; 2011. 549p

[2] Miranda GMD, Mendes ACG, da Silva AL. Population aging in Brazil: Current and future social challenges and consequences. Revista Brasileira de Geriatria e Gerontologia. 2016;**19**(3):507-519. DOI: 10.1590/1809-98232016019.150140

[3] Lapão LV, Arcênio RA, Popolin MP, Rodrigues LBB. The role of Primary Healthcare in the coordination of Health Care Networks in Rio de Janeiro, Brazil, and Lisbon region, Portugal. Ciência & Saúde Coletiva. 2017;**22**(3):713-723. DOI: 10.1590/1413-81232017223.33532016

[4] Arruda C, Lopes SGR, Koerich MHAL, Winck DR, Meirelles BHS, de Mello ALSF. Health care networks under the light of the complexity theory. Escola Anna Nery. 2015;**19**(1):169-173. DOI: 10.5935/1414-8145.20150023

[5] Ministério da Saúde-Brasil. Portaria nº 4.279, de 30 de dezembro de 2010. Estabelece diretrizes para a organização da Rede de Atenção à Saúde no âmbito do Sistema Único de Saúde (SUS). Brasília: Ministério da Saúde; 2010

[6] Ministério da Saúde-Brasil, Conselho Nacional de Secretários de Saúde. A Atenção Primária e as Redes de Atenção à Saúde. Brasília: CONASS; 2015

[7] Viegas APB, Carmo RF, Luz ZMP. Fatores que influenciam o acesso aos serviços de saúde na visão de profissionais e usuários de uma unidade básica de referência. Saúde e Sociedade. 2015;**24**(1):100-112. DOI: 10.1590/S0104-12902015000100008

[8] Mendes EV. As redes de atenção à saúde. Ciência & Saúde Coletiva. 2010;**15**(5):2297-2305. DOI: 10.1590/S1413-81232010000500005

[9] Moll MF, Goulart MB, Caprio AP, Ventura CAA, Ogoshi AACM. The knowledge of nurses on health care networks. Journal of Nursing UFPE on line. 2017;**11**(1):86-93. DOI: 10.5205/reuol.9978-88449-6-1101201711

[10] Atty ATM, Tomazelli JG. Palliative care in home care for cancer patients in Brazil. Saúde e Debate. 2018;**42**(116):225-236. DOI: 10.1590/0103-1104201811618

[11] Manchola C, Brazão E, Pulschen A, Santos M. Palliative care, spirituality and narrative bioethics in a Specialized Health Care Unit. Revista Bioética. 2016;**24**(1):165-175

[12] Clos MB, Grossi PK. Desafios para o cuidado digno em instituições de longa permanência. Revista Bioética. 2016;**24**(2):395-406. DOI: 10.1590/1983-80422016241118

[13] Academia Nacional de Cuidados Paliativos (ANCP). Panorama dos Cuidados Paliativos no Brasil. São Paulo: ANCP; 2018. 15p

[14] Frossard A. Os cuidados paliativos como política pública: Notas introdutórias. Cadernos EBAPE. BR. 2016;**14**(spe):640-655. DOI: 10.1590/1679-395114315

[15] Gomes ALZ, Othero MB. Cuidados paliativos. Estudos Avançados. 2016;**30**(88):155-166. DOI: 10.1590/S0103-40142016.30880011

[16] Alves RF, Andrade SFO, Melo MO, Cavalcante KB, Angelim RM. Cuidados paliativos: Desafios para cuidadores e profissionais de saúde. Fractal: Revista de Psicologia. 2015;**27**(2):165-176. DOI: 10.1590/1984-0292/943

[17] Morosini L. Cuidados paliativos: Qualidade de vida. Revista Radis Comunicação e Saúde. 2016;**168**:12

[18] World Health Organization (WHO). Cancer Pain Relief and Palliative Care, Geneva, Technical Report Series. Geneva: World Health Organization; 1990

[19] World Health Organization (WHO). The Solid Facts: Palliative Care. Copenhagen: WHO Regional Office for Europe. Geneva: World Health Organization; 2004

[20] Gomomez BX, Martinez M, Blay C, Amblas J, Villanueuva A, Costa X, et al. Identifying patients with chronic conditions in need of palliative care in the general population: Development of the NECPAL tool and preliminary prevalence rates in Catalonia. BMJ Supportive & Palliative Care. 2013;**3**(3):300-308. DOI: 10.1136/bmjspcare-2012-000211

[21] Instituto Nacional de Câncer (INCA). História do INCA [Internet]. Available from: http://www.inca.gov.br/conteudo_view.asp?id=235

[22] de Paiva FCL, de Almeida Júnior JJ, Damásio AC. Ética em cuidados paliativos: Concepções sobre o fim da vida. Revista Bioética. 2014;**22**(3):550-560. DOI: 10.1590/1983-80422014223038

[23] Vasconcelos GB, Pereira PM. Cuidados paliativos em atenção domiciliar: Uma revisão bibliográfica. Revista de Administração em Saúde. 2018;**18**(70). DOI: 10.23973/ras.70.85

[24] Ministério da Saúde-Brasil. Resolução n° 41/GM de 31 de Outubro de 2018. Dispõe Sobre as Diretrizes Para a Organização dos Cuidados Paliativos, à Luz dos Cuidados Continuados Integrados, no Âmbito Sistema Único de Saúde (SUS). Brasília: Diário Oficial da União; 2018. Sec. 1:276

[25] World Health Organization (WHO). Integrating Palliative Care and Symptom Relief into Primary Health Care: A WHO Guide for Planners, Implementers and Managers. Geneva: World Health Organization; 2018

[26] World Health Organization (WHO). Palliative care. In: Cancer Control: Knowledge Into Action: WHO Guide for Effective Programs. Module 05. WHO Library; Genève: 2007

[27] Braz MS, Franco MHP. Profissionais paliativistas e suas contribuições na prevenção de luto complicado. Psicologia: Ciência e Profissão. 2017;**37**(1):90-105. DOI: 10.1590/1982-3703001702016

[28] World Health Organization (WHO). Definição de Cuidados Paliativos da WHO [Internet]. GENEVA. 2017. Available from: https://www.who.int/palliativecare/en/

[29] Gomes B, Higginson IJ, Calanzani N, Cohen J, Deliens L, Daveson BA, et al. Preferences for place of death if faced with advanced cancer: A population survey in England, Flanders, Germany, Italy, the Netherlands, Portugal and Spain. Annals of Oncology. 2012;**23**(8):2006-2015. DOI: 10.1093/annonc/mdr602

[30] Carvalho GAFL, de Menezes RMP, Enders BC, Teixeira GA, Dantas DNA, de Oliveira DRC.Meanings attributed to palliative care by health professional in the primary care context. Texto & Contexto Enfermagem. 2018;**27**(2):e5740016. DOI: 10.1590/0104-070720180005740016

[31] Mc Namara B, Rosenwax LK, Holman CDJ. A method for defining and estimating the palliative care population. Journal of Pain and Symptom Management. 2006;**32**(1):5-12. DOI: 10.1016/j.jpainsymman.2005.12.018

[32] Smith S, Brick A, O'Hara S, Normand C. Evidence on the cost and cost-effectiveness of palliative care: A literature review. Palliative Medicine. 2014;**28**(2):130-150. DOI: 10.1177/0269216313493466

[33] Savassi LCM. Os atuais desafios da Atenção Domiciliar na Atenção Primária à Saúde: Uma análise na perspectiva do Sistema Único de Saúde. Revista Brasileira de Medicina de Família e Comunidade. 2016;**11**(38):1-12. DOI: 10.5712/rbmfc11(38)1259

[34] Ministério da Saúde-Brasil. Portaria n° 963/GM de 27 de maio de 2013. Redefine a Atenção Domiciliar no âmbito do Sistema Único de Saúde (SUS). Brasília: Diário Oficial da União; 2013. Sec. 1:30

[35] dos Santos Junior AG, Santos FR dos Pessalacia JDR. Challenges for hospice care in primary health care: Integrative review literature. Journal of Nursing UFPE on line. 2016;**10**(7):2708-2719. DOI: 10.5205/reuol.9106-80230-1-SM1007201650

[36] Ernesto SA, Duarte ED. Cuidado paliativo na atenção domiciliar: Conhecimento, definição e elegibilidade na perspectiva do profissional de saúde. In: XVI Coloquio Panamericano de Investigación en Enfermería; 2018

[37] Malagutti W, Roehrs H. A Legislação e os cuidados paliativos no Brasil. In: Silva RS, Amaral JB, Malagutti W, editors. Enfermagem em Cuidados Paliativos, Cuidando Para Uma boa Morte. 4th ed. São Paulo: Martinari; 2019. p. 93

[38] Pereira BS, Tomase E. Instrumento de apoio à gestão regional de saúde para monitoramento de indicadores de saúde. Epidemiologia e Serviços de Saúde. 2016;**25**(2):411-418. DOI: 10.5123/s1679-49742016000200019

[39] Garcia JBS, Rodrigues RF, Limas SF. A estruturação de um serviço de cuidados paliativos no Brasil: Relato de experiência. Revista Brasileira de Anestesiologia. 2014;**64**(4):286-291. DOI: 10.1016/j.bjan.2013.06.007

Chapter 7

Palliative Care: The Nigerian Perspective

Nnadi Daniel Chukwunyere

Abstract

Palliative care is an area of healthcare that focuses on relieving and preventing the suffering of patients. It utilizes a multidisciplinary team approach to ensure a "holistic" care of the patient. It is a relatively new concept in medicine and the Nigerian experience has not been widely studied. Despite its introduction into the nation over two decades ago, it still faces a lot of challenges in terms of integration into the health care system, implementation and governmental policy. With increasing longevity, urbanization, high prevalence of HIV/AIDS and chronic diseases including malignancies, there will be an increasing number of Nigerians requiring palliative care.

Keywords: palliative care, holistic approach, Nigeria

1. Introduction

When treatment for cure is not possible and the only option is palliative, the patient is said to be terminally ill [3]. In a patient that is terminally ill, the estimated life expectancy is less than or equal to 6 months, under the assumption that the disease will run its natural course [3, 2].

Care of the terminally ill, infirm and elderly individuals has been a key part of many societies. Since the fourth century, Rest house, Sarai, Sanatorium and Hot springs, were developed as special places to attend to their needs [1–3]. It has been realized that the needs of terminally ill patients were not met by the then prevailing specialist or non-specialist health system. Terminal care was not as elaborate as it is performed today. It was initially carried out by nuns and other charitable organizations. Palliative care was not included in the existing health care system of those days. Individuals and groups with a Christian commitment have been important in establishing pioneering palliative care programs in many places, and again have usually seen in education the best hope of contributing to care for the dying. From the 1980s rapid progress was made in developing palliative care as a discipline in the health care delivery.

The word "palliative" in Latin means "caring" [1]. This is the total care of patients whose conditions do not respond to curative treatment. It relieves suffering and improves the quality of life for both patients and families throughout an illness experience, not just at the end of life. Sometimes palliative care and hospice care are confused, and they have similar goals. However, hospice care is specifically for terminally ill patients while palliative care is more general and offered to patients whose conditions are not necessarily terminal. Palliative care begins when illness is diagnosed and continues regardless of whether the patient receives treatment directed at the disease.

IntechOpen

According to the World Health Organization (WHO), palliative care is defined as "an approach that improves the quality of life of patients and their families facing the problem associated with life-threatening illness, through the prevention and relief of suffering by means of early identification and impeccable assessment and treatment of pain and other problems, physical, psycho-social and spiritual" [1]. It is the comprehensive care of the individual whose is considered as having a body, soul, spirit and family members who require support. It is also about living as well as dying with dignity. It is a good practice for the physician to refer his patients who require palliative care to access such care. This will not necessarily diminish our status as health care providers. Palliative care is often referred to as end-of-life care, but when properly carried out, it has been found to improve outcomes of patients with terminal diseases even leading to increased survival. The focus is not on death, but on compassionate specialized care for the living. Most health services are designed for prevention, diagnosis and treatment of diseases, but there is a huge need for ongoing care those who do not get better.

Palliative care is usually an organized care, which can be given, in a hospital setting, hospice or in the home of the patients. Resource constraints in developing countries, direct the site of care. Home-based care is cheap and acceptable to the family and the patient, and can offer care that respects cultural practice and removes the need for family attendance at hospital [4, 5].

The approach to patients care is "holistic," meaning that the patient is viewed as a person with physical, psychological, social and cultural gifts and needs which are special to that person [4]. The holistic approach looks after problems in four groups:

1. Physical: symptoms

2. Psychological: worries, fears, sadness, anger

3. Social: family needs, issues of food, work, housing and relationships

4. Spiritual: questions of meaning of life and death, the need to be at peace

It thus involves a multi-professional team approach. This is a team of professionals who are committed to working together to provide the patient and her family comprehensive care. Palliative care is "a calling." The team must be prepared to offer selfless service without expecting reward and function as a family, showing love for each other and those who visit them—patients, relations, and visitors. Recognize that every member of the team is precious. Volunteers are expected to attend a course to allow them see the depth of hospice care. Confidentiality and ethical issues are a priority.

The pioneering works of Dame Cicely Saunders in the United Kingdom and of Anne Merriman in Africa drew the attention of the medical community and the public to the evolution of palliative care in the 1960s [1, 6]. In the African continent, Uganda, South Africa and Kenya are among the earliest to develop palliative care. In November 2002, in Cape Town South Africa, the African palliative care association (APCA) was formed [7]. It was registered in 2003 and opened its headquarters in Uganda in 2005 as a non-governmental organization (NGO), with a regional mandate to promote and scale-up culturally appropriate and affordable palliative care for people with progressive, life-threatening and life-limiting illness. Palliative care is still at a developmental stage in Nigeria despite decades of its introduction by Mrs. Fatunmbi and Dr. Anne Merriman in Nigeria in 1993 [8]. The year 2003 was when palliative care was properly introduced to the Nigerian government, policy-makers and general public. It is now known as the Center for Palliative Care Nigeria

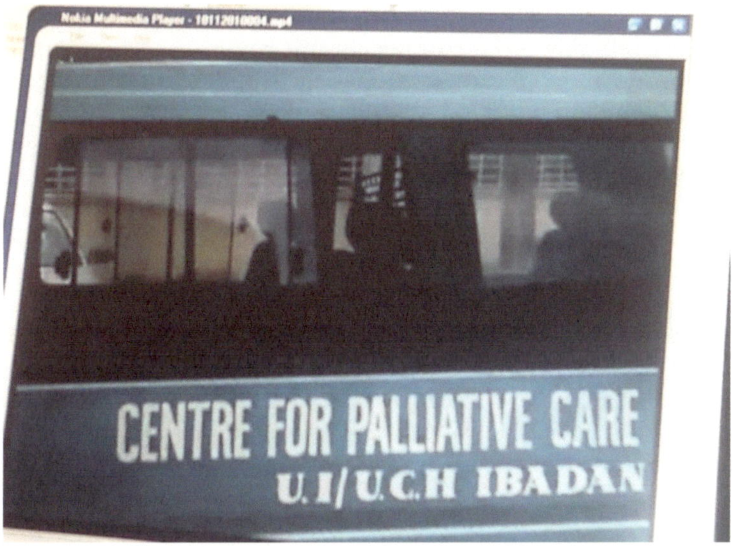

Figure 1.
The center for palliative care at the University College Hospital (UCH), Ibadan. It provides day care and outreach services for home-based care.

(CPCN), located at the University College Hospital (UCH), Ibadan [8]. In 2007, CPCN launched its day-care hospice within the UCH as shown in **Figure 1**. A pain and palliative care unit was established in 2008 at the multidisciplinary oncology center of the University of Nigeria in Enugu, South-eastern Nigeria [9].

2. Palliative care in Nigeria

Nigeria is the most populous country in Africa. It has an estimated population of 160–180 million scattered around six geopolitical zones and 774 local government areas (LGA). The country has the third largest number of people living with HIV/AIDS after South Africa and India [10]. Approximately 100,000 new cases of cancer occur annually in Nigeria and thus there are large numbers of patients needing palliative care [9]. There is a gradual erosion of the hitherto extended family support and patients get isolated both at home and in the hospitals. The life expectancy is lower than in most of the developed countries with low gross domestic product (GDP). The annual national budget for health is a ridiculous 1.5–3%, oscillating whenever there is a change in Government. Medical services are provided through out-pocket payment or user fees. Health insurance is provided mainly to the 1% of the population employed in the civil service. Thus, provision of adequate health services goes to the highest bidder.

Palliative care is still new to the country owing to the fact that it is not included as an area of specialization for health professionals across the country. It is now currently offered as an undergraduate course at the College of Medicine, University of Ibadan and postgraduate diploma in a privately owned University in Ilorin, Kwara state [8].

In 2006, Dr. Oyebola Folaju, became the first specialist in palliative medicine in Nigeria following a postgraduate training in palliative medicine at the famous University of Cape Town, South Africa [8]. He pioneered palliative medicine in Nigeria and became the first full-time pain and palliative care physician by establishing the first pain and palliative medicine department at the Federal Medical

Centre Abeokuta, Nigeria. This was the first hospital-based palliative medicine services and the beginning of integrating chronic pain management, palliative and end-of-life care, into an acute care hospital in the country [8]. Through his efforts the country today can boast of more than 15 similar facilities in Nigeria making use of their local institutional policies to move forward. Most families prefer the home-based care. It provides familiar environment, opportunity to attend to siblings, access to family and friends and privacy are advantages. This is performed in conjunction with family, primary care team and specialist within the hospital or hospice.

Despite the prescriptions of the WHO in 2002 and its re-emphasize at the 2004 WHO general assembly that palliative care should be integrated into all nations' health care system, several African countries including Nigeria are yet to approve it as a policy. This situation had contributed significantly to the slow level of palliative care development in Nigeria, as the palliative care practitioners have no access to the nation health budget.

3. Palliative care-challenges in Nigeria

The problems militating against the provision of palliative care in Nigeria can be broadly classified into the following:

1. Poor awareness, knowledge and skills

2. Inability to discuss cancer diagnosis and management with patients

3. Lack of trained professionals

4. Lack of resources

5. Problems associated with availability of medications including oral opioids

6. Lack of government policy/priority

3.1 Poor awareness

In Nigeria, 60–70% of patients present to health care facilities with advanced disease, when treatment for cure is virtually impossible [11–13]. Patients are referred late for care and by the time they get to the palliative care center, most of them were already down. The reasons for late presentation include late recognition of initial symptoms due to lack of knowledge, search for alternate treatment and cure, inappropriate advice, poverty and fear of hospitals. Such patients at presentation are at an advanced stage of the disease with several distressing symptoms requiring palliative care.

Many victims of terminal diseases have died as a result of lack of knowledge about palliative care. Statistical data are grossly inadequate and unreliable in Nigeria. The absence of a population-based cancer registry in the country has hampered policy formulation and planning [7]. In a study about knowledge of palliative among medical interns in a tertiary health institution in north-west Nigeria by Nnadi and Singh in 2016, the interns showed inadequate knowledge about palliative care. Among those that reported knowledge about palliative care, many held misconceptions regarding the signs and symptoms and the disease conditions that require palliative care [14]. The sources of knowledge about palliative care were mainly from school lectures and healthcare personnel. This underscores the need to include palliative care in the school curriculum both at the undergraduate and postgraduate levels. The residency training is a critical window of opportunity for training about good end-of-life care for dying patients and their relatives [14].

A similar study in Ibadan, Nigeria in 2002 on the knowledge and attitudes of terminally ill patients and their relatives to palliative care and hospice services in Nigeria, showed gross lack of knowledge about palliative care in our community, but a positive attitude towards palliative and hospice services [4].

There is also poor knowledge of palliative care among health care workers and reluctance by doctors in Nigeria to prescribe morphine where it is available because of fear of addiction. Morphine remains a controlled drug in Nigeria and in some other countries because of fear of diversion of prescribed morphine. Knowledge gap have also been identified even among health care practitioners that provide palliative care in terms of their understanding of the goals that palliative care seeks to achieve [15]. Financial constraint is given as the major physical factor that prevents the patients from acquiring even their pain medications.

3.2 Spiritual consciousness

Nigeria is a multi-ethnic, multicultural and multi-religious country. Islam is the major religion in the north, while Christianity predominates in the south. In between there is an amalgamation of Christianity and Islamic religious practices. Despite the practice of these major religions, traditional religious worship reign supreme. The influence of traditional religion permeates the life of an average Nigerian. Religion influences our action, our decision, inspirations, goals, motivations, principles and our contentment. Thus traditional medicine practitioners are well patronized and are usually the first port of call especially in the rural setting. Orthodox medical care is still viewed with suspicion even among the educated class.

There is a belief in a diabolical interference existent in almost all illnesses in Nigeria. Accusing fingers are usually pointed to an "envious" neighbor or mate as being responsible even for the slightest form of ill health. The rising trend of the Pentecostal religious movement has not helped matters. It poses a significant means of spiritual or faith-based healing among Nigerians. The health implication is that among many Nigerian Christians, faith healing ministers have taken the place of conventional therapists for their health problems. These confirm that the belief in the efficacy of African traditional healing and church spiritual healing is so strong among Nigerians that they rely on these methods irrespective of some experiences of failures. Thus, many individuals who are unfortunate to be befallen by terminal diseases, attribute their predicaments to witchcraft and spiritual attacks [9].

Many Nigerians don't believe in making their wills until the final moment because of a strong belief in dying by natural means and for fear of being killed by disaffected family members. Thus speaking of impending death is seen as a taboo. This presents a major obstacle in rendering palliative care in our environment. There seems to be a culture of "death denial" among patients, their relatives, and healthcare professionals [16]. Thus having an eye-to-eyeball discussion of impending death with a terminally ill patient may result in stigmatization of the doctor. Suspicion, abuse, rejection of therapy and even signing against medical advice may follow. The patient may then gravitate from one health care facility to another in a futile attempt to get cure. Spiritual homes, faith-based healing centers and herbal remedies would be profusely patronized at a great cost to the patient. When eventually death comes, the family and dependents are left impoverished and unable to foot the burial expenses. Our people hardly accept the reality of failed treatment or death. Their firm belief is that doctors treat and make patients well. The doctor must continue to offer hope even when reality is to the contrary. Where death is accepted, many would want to be at home so that they can make their peace, say farewell, and give final instructions to immediate relatives [9]. Hence one finds that many terminally ill keep away from medical treatment for fear of hospitalization.

3.3 Psycho-social problems

The model approach to palliative care in the western world differs significantly from the African setting. Palliative care needs in African countries include home and respite care, pain and symptom control, financial, emotional and spiritual support, and also food, shelter, legal help, and school fees. Management of disease-related pain in patients with hunger pains highlights the importance of adapting palliative care models from developing countries to African settings. Traditions dictate appropriate models and places of care: sick people might be removed from villages to avoid risk to the community, or returned from the hospital to the community to avoid dangers of overcrowded wards and toxic drugs from developed countries. Access to effective cancer pain relief is hampered by poor social conditions, criminality and urban violence.

There is some social stigma associated with disease entities. Stigma can prevent patients with HIV/AIDS from referring themselves to palliative care.

Many Nigerians would not want to be associated with terminal diseases. They believe that if the public comes to know about their state of health, it would bring dishonor to them and family [9]. The stigmatization that is being shown to victims of deadly diseases in Nigeria, affects the socio-economic progress of the country, as the sufferers probably miss work, and are unemployed or stop-working early. In the mainly Islamic northern part of the country, cultural norms such as Purdah restrictions can prevent women from seeking health care outside the home for themselves. Cultural norms such as traditional practices and use of herbs also discourage the use of more effective modern medical practices. This underscores the relevance of social support in coping with adversity among patients of diverse ethnic origin. In Nigeria, the perception of ill-health is much more complex than the mainstream biomedical approach. The concept of well-being and ill-health is much more holistic, involving the body, the mind and in some instances the supernatural. Thus, superstition, ignorance and cultural practices tend to affect the health-seeking behavior of our people. In our setting, the multidisciplinary palliative care team should include spiritual care givers, family members and friends so as to meet the entire needs of the patient.

3.4 Governmental policy

Palliative care in Nigeria is still at a developmental stage. Initially the attitude of the Nigerian government towards palliative care was weak and non-committal due to lack of advocacy. Through the efforts of the Hospice and palliative care association of Nigeria (HPCAN), palliative care services have appreciated in almost all the six geopolitical zones of the country. The association has liaised with the federal ministry of health to establish palliative care units in all tertiary health institutions in the country. In addition, the federal government of Nigeria has designated six federal hospitals as oncology centers of excellence.

Despite all these, there remain a lot of challenges in implementation of effective palliative care services in Nigeria. Many cancer treatment centers are located mainly in the urban setting. Thus patients in the rural areas cannot access them due to distance barriers and poverty. Many radiotherapy centers in the country lack functional machines. Even when the machines are available, there is dearth of adequate manpower to maintain them. Morphine, the gold standard medication for pain relief in cancer patients, remains a controlled drug in Nigeria. Due to fear of misuse and abuse, the government is yet to decentralize the distribution of opioids in the country. The Federal Ministry of Health remains the sole importer of opioids, while the National Agency for Food and Drug Administration and Control (NAFDAC) monitors the distribution. The result is that morphine is not readily available to those that need it [8, 9]. Some health workers consequently, have resorted to less effective but more available alternative medications such as Tramadol and Pentazocine, for pain relief.

The problems facing the implementation of effective palliative care in Nigeria cannot be excised from the overall prevailing socio-economic condition in the country. Poverty, ignorance, insecurity, poor funding of healthcare, inadequate manpower and poor policy formulation and implementation constitute obstacles to effective good health care delivery.

4. The way forwards

There is a paucity of information on hospice and palliative care provision in Nigeria and only a weak evidence base upon which to build policy and practice development. Overall, services remain scattered and piecemeal in the country, and coverage is poor. Pioneer workers in palliative care established small models of care to act as foci for education initiatives, so that palliative care can spread to wider areas. They saw in education, as the best hope of contributing care for the dying. It would be wishful thinking to assume that age old beliefs could be eradicated in a twinkle of the eye, but education will create awareness, remove taboos, and modify some attitudes and behaviors. The best way to do this is by incorporating palliative care into the medical undergraduate curriculum and residency training program. Public enlightenment through the print and electronic media will further create awareness; eliminate the stigma associated with terminal illness and regard dying as a normal process. It will provide psycho-social, spiritual and bereavement support for family members. Patients with terminal diseases should be encouraged to seek palliative care at a place best suitable for them. Outreach services for home-based care should be encouraged and adequately funded.

We need advocacy to present our case to the general populace. Government alone cannot shoulder the responsibility involved in implementing an effective palliative care. The private sector of the economy, corporate bodies, religious and traditional leaders need to be carried along. The government needs to address its policy on availability and distribution of morphine in the country. Palliative care champions in Nigeria are working to demonstrate how morphine access can be appropriately integrated into healthcare systems. Through political advocacy and public awareness, the necessity of integrated palliative care can be better understood.

5. Conclusion

Both Specialist and integrated palliative care have important role in Nigeria as the "extended family" system is fast breaking down. Grafting palliative care into existing networks of home-based care is feasible and must be adapted to Nigerian needs. Government policy and support, private-public partnership initiative, collaboration with partners is essential to establish palliative care education and service in Nigeria. Palliative care is all about love, support, care, effective control of pain and distressing symptoms in times of special needs.

Acknowledgements

We acknowledge the previous author cited in the text.

Conflict of interest

Nil declared.

Author details

Nnadi Daniel Chukwunyere
Department of Obstetrics and Gynaecology, Usmanu Danfodiyo University Teaching Hospital, Sokoto, Nigeria

*Address all correspondence to: dc.nnadi@gmail.com

References

[1] Goldstein M, Houtepen R, Proot IM, Abu-Saad HH, Spreeuweberg C, et al. What is a good death? Terminally ill patients: Dealing with normative expectations around death and dying. Patient Education and Counseling. 2006;**64**:378-386

[2] Kulkami PD. Hospital-based palliative care: A case for integrating care with cure. Indian Journal of Palliative Care. 2011;**17**:74-76

[3] WHO. WHO Definition of Palliative Care [Internet]. Available from: http://www.who.int/cancer/palliative/definition/en/ [Accessed: September 19, 2010]

[4] Adenikpekun A, Onibokun A, Elumelu TN, SOA. Knowledge and attitudes of terminally-ill patients and their families to palliative care and hospice services in Nigeria. Nigerian Journal of Clinical Practice. 2005;**8**(1):19-22

[5] Maltoni M, Nanni O, Naldoni M. Evaluation of cost of home therapy for patients with terminal disease. Current opinion in oncology. 1998;**10**(4):302-309

[6] Merriman A. In the darkness of the shadow of death: A ray of hope: The story of hospice Africa. Journal of Palliative Care. 1993;**9**(3):23-24

[7] Shambe IH. Palliative care in Nigeria: Challenges and prospects. Jos Journal of Medicine. 2014;**8**(3):53-55

[8] Oyebola FO. Palliative care trends and challenges in Nigeria—The journey so far. International Journal of Emergency Medicine. 2017;**1**(2):17

[9] Onyeka TC. Palliative care in Enugu, Nigeria: Challenges to a new practice. Indian Journal of Palliative Care. 2011;**17**(2):131-136

[10] Akinwande O, Ogundiran T, Akarolo-Anthony S, Mamadu I, Dakum P, Blattner W, et al. Challenges in treating malignancies in HIV in Nigeria. Current Opinion in Oncology. 2009;**21**:455-461

[11] Soyannwu OA. Cancer pain–progress and ongoing issues in Africa. Pain Research & Management. 2009;**14**:349

[12] Adenipekun A, Onibokun A, Elumelu TN, Soyannwo OA. Knowledge and attitudes of terminally ill patients and their family to palliative care and hospice services in Nigeria. Nigerian Journal of Clinical Practice. 2005;**8**:19-22

[13] Olaitan S, Oladayo A, Ololade M. Palliative care: Supporting adult cancer patients in Ibadan, Nigeria. Journal of Palliative Care and Medicine. 2016;**6**:258. DOI: 10.4172/2165-7386.1000258

[14] Nnadi DC, Singh S. Knowledge about palliative care among medical interns in a tertiary health institution in Northwestern Nigeria. Indian Journal of Palliative Care. 2016;**22**:343-347

[15] Fadare JO, Obimakinde AM, Olaogun DO, Afolayan JN. Perception of nurses about palliative care: Experience from south-West Nigeria. Annals of Medical and Health Sciences Research. 2014;**4**:723-727

[16] Odimegwu O. Perils of operating palliative care in Nigeria. Available from: www.modernghana.com/news/471174/1/Nigeria. [Accessed: 3 Jun, 2013]

Chapter 8

Palliative Care Services from Past to Present

Murat Can Mollaoğlu, Döne Günay and Mukadder Mollaoğlu

Abstract

Palliative care (PC) refers to all services provided to make the remaining life of a patient meaningful and valuable. It is recommended that palliative care that is applied to improve the life quality of the patients should not be based only on the diagnosis and prognosis of the disease but also on the need of the patients. Even, palliative care was administered only in the late stages of diseases in the past, but these days it is recommended to be administered in addition to therapies starting from the diagnosis of life-threatening diseases. Palliative care requires a multidisciplinary team approach consisting of professionals who serve for a common purpose. No single palliative care model can be fit for all conditions. However, there is a universal fundamental principle of palliative care: it should address the individual wishes and needs of each patient and the relatives of patients. The development and training of palliative care services vary from country to country: palliative care services are in the development stage in developing countries, compared to developed countries. This chapter provides necessary information about palliative care services, a multidisciplinary health service.

Keywords: palliative care, the purpose of palliative care, palliative care models, palliative care levels, palliative care in the world

1. Introduction

Scientific and medical advances in the last century have prolonged and facilitated life and delayed death. Advances in biomedical and clinical medicine have enabled the prevention and/or treatment of many diseases [1]. Recently, improvements in treatment models have significantly reduced or palliated the crucial effect of many diseases which were killing people in a short time in the past [2].

The World Health Organization (WHO) defined palliative care for the first time in 1989 as follows: "palliative care is an approach that improves the life quality of patients and their families facing the problem associated with life-threatening illness, through the prevention and relief of suffering by means of early identification and impeccable assessment and treatment of pain and other problems, physical, psychosocial and spiritual" [3]. In 2014, the WHO added another view to the definition: "Palliative care is the responsibility of all physicians"; thus, the definition of palliative care became comprehensive [4, 5]. Palliative care is a multidisciplinary care that aims to prevent or palliate the symptoms, *relief of suffering of patients*, and improve life quality of them [6]. Palliative care should not only be applied to patients in the final stages of life: it should be integrated into medical care and curative and life-long treatment, regardless of disease stage

[7, 8]. In palliative care, patient-specific care, family support, multidisciplinary teamwork, and effective communication are essential [6]. In short, palliative care is a philosophy of care and is based on holistic care and support for families including the mourning period [9, 10].

2. Purpose, philosophy, and components of palliative care

2.1 The purpose of palliative care

The goal of palliative care is to restore the functional capacity of a patient by being sensitive to the cultural and local values, beliefs, and practices of the individual, to alleviate pain, and to improve the life quality by controlling the symptoms [6, 11, 12]. In other words, the purpose is to reduce or eliminate the symptoms of the disease without any further examinations when the cure is no longer possible in the disease. Indeed, what the WHO expected from palliative care team is to respect patients and their relatives and to consider their wishes. This expectation should be interpreted as providing health care to the patient and his/her relatives that will ensure their well-being regardless of their age, economic or social status, and disease characteristics [1, 4, 7, 9, 13].

2.2 Basic principles of palliative care

The basic principles of palliative care can be summarized as follows:

- To integrate the psychosocial and spiritual aspects of patient care
- To reduce other symptoms, pain in the first place
- To ensure that the patient and the relatives of the patient accept death as a normal process
- To neither expedite nor delay death
- To make the patient as active as possible until death
- To provide support to patients' relatives to cope with problems during the illness
- To identify and meet the needs of the patient and his/her family including the mourning period
- To manage the clinical complications resulting from treatments such as radiotherapy and chemotherapy [7, 9, 14, 15]

2.3 Philosophy of palliative care

According to the philosophy of palliative care, the patients are provided with care and support in various institutions; death is part of ordinary life; physical, social, and spiritual aspects of care all are integrated; and the main targets are to enhanced life quality of the patients and to ensure that the patient quickly returns to his/her social life [10, 16].

Cancer patients in need of palliative care are a group of patients with high psychosocial, spiritual, and physical needs who experience many different symptoms, especially pain [6, 8]. In addition, the level of distress experienced by the family and its members increases in this period, and this situation affects the family order intensively. The most common problems experienced by cancer patients include physical symptoms such as pain, nausea, vomiting, fatigue, constipation, and loss of appetite. However, psychological problems such as anxiety, fear, helplessness, hopelessness, exhaustion, and depression are also common in patients. Economic and social problems are other important problems for cancer patients [6, 8, 10, 13]. Patients' need for palliative care to cope with all these problems is increasing. Palliative care includes a holistic approach to cancer treatment that can improve or optimize the quality of life of cancer patients and their relatives in the best possible way, meeting the needs [4, 6, 9].

Palliative care is one of the most critical building blocks of the war against cancer. Palliative care is a significant health service, responsibility, medical requirement, and need from the diagnosis of cancer to the end of life and is an indispensable element of national health policies. Therefore, it is imperative that the palliative care service for cancer patients has basic dimensions such as symptom control; psychological, spiritual, and emotional support; support for the families and relatives of cancer patients; and support during the mourning period [4, 7, 13]. The World Health Organization envisages the development of palliative care services in all countries. The WHO also envisions the establishment of a palliative care service network, which can serve the whole country, in underdeveloped countries with low-income levels even if they can do nothing about cancer [7]. The WHO recommends the completion of shortcomings in palliative care, rather than the investments that could bring considerable burdens on the country's economy, such as expensive treatments, radiotherapy devices, or screening programs [1, 5].

2.4 Palliative care team

Palliative care is provided by a team of experienced and trained medical staff who serve for a common purpose and volunteer. This service needs multidisciplinary healthcare services, including an algologist, oncologist, neurologist, surgeon, palliative care nurse, cleric, social volunteers, and psychologist [10, 17].

Besides what is mentioned, it also needs an interdisciplinary approach; the palliative care team provides care to the patient and his/her family and plans the care plan to include the various components according to the current and future needs of the patient [17, 18].

These components are listed as follows:

Patient population: palliative care is for patients in all age groups who are affected by chronic illness or trauma and whose life quality is adversely affected [12, 17].

Patient- and family-oriented care: in palliative care, the patient and his family should be given tailored care, and the care plan should be applied and evaluated individually taking into account the patient's and family's preferences and objectives [8, 17].

The continuity of palliative care: palliative care should start with the diagnosis of a life-threatening disease and should continue throughout the treatment period, after treatment, and until the death of the individual and during the mourning period [6, 17].

Comprehensive care: in palliative care, multidimensional diagnosis is required to eliminate the psychological, spiritual, social, and physical problems of the individual and his/her family and to alleviate pain [4, 17].

Interdisciplinary team: a palliative care team should primarily include medical, nursing, and social work professionals. Palliative care may also require a broad team of collaborators, such as psychologists, pharmacologists, religious officials, mourning consultants, dietitian, physics/vocational/art/game and music therapists, case managers, trained volunteers, home care assistants, and voluntary organizations [7, 17].

Alleviation of the pain: the primary objective of palliative care is to take measures to prevent the pain and other symptoms, as well as the many problems caused by the disease and treatment, and to eliminate these problems [6, 17].

Communication skills: effective communication in palliative care is crucial for helping to make medical decisions, determining goals and preferences, active listening, and sharing of useful information.

The skill of care during death and mourning period: in the process of mourning and loss, the palliative care team must be aware of the age-related physical and psychosocial symptoms, the care and support needs of the patient and his family, the early signs and symptoms of death, and the prognosis of death [8, 17].

Ensuring continuity of care between institutions: palliative care should work in conjunction with all systems involved in health care (such as hospitals, emergency services, hospices, home care, community, and school). The palliative care team should cooperate with professional and nongovernmental organizations in these specified healthcare settings to ensure the continuity and coordination of palliative care [17, 18].

Equality in accessing palliative care: the palliative care team is responsible for providing a service that is accessible to all, regardless of race, ethnicity, gender, socioeconomic status, place of residence, and cultural attitudes [12, 17].

Quality service delivery: palliative care services should be of high quality and outstanding. It is vital to regularly determine the requirements for a quality service, to measure the care process using appropriate measurement tools, and to ensure continuity [4, 8, 10, 17].

2.5 Palliative care needs

Palliative care provides a cost-effective service by reducing unnecessary diagnostic and therapeutic interventions, ineffective intensive care, and emergency department admissions [14, 19]. It has been reported that the integration of palliative care from the early stages of the disease increases the quality of care and prolongs the life span [18, 20].

Patients, who are bedbound, do not have curative treatment and have difficulty in controlling physical and emotional symptoms evaluated by the palliative care team. If the palliative care team thinks that it will improve the life quality of the patient and his/her family, the patient is admitted to the palliative care unit [19, 21].

Criteria for admission to palliative care unit:

1. Patients with a visual analogue scale (VAS) pain score of ≥5 despite medical treatment, impaired sleep patterns due to pain, and persistent pain even at rest and patients that cannot be administered with medical treatment due to side effects

2. Malnutrition patients whose oral intake is impaired, who have a nutritional risk screening 2002 score of ≥3, have a weight loss over 10% in the last 6 months, and who need enteral or parenteral nutrition because they cannot feed orally

3. Patients who is infected and treatment-resistant and who has stage III–IV (according to Norton/Braden) decubitus ulcer

4. Patients who are diagnosed with delirium and whose etiology is multiple or uncertain

5. Geriatric syndromes: falls, incontinence, neglect, and abuse

6. Fragile patients with treatment-resistant stage IV heart failure

7. Patients with worsening clinical symptoms and laboratory symptoms (dyspnea, hemoptysis, uncontrolled pain, etc.) despite treatment; patients with a Karnofsky Performance Scale score of <70%; patients with oncological emergencies such as vertebra metastasis and hypercalcemia; patients who had pneumonia more than two times in the last 3 months; oncology patients with high comorbidity, shorter life expectancy than 6 months, and progressive disease despite treatments such as surgery, radiotherapy, and chemotherapy

8. Patients with treatment-resistant end-stage chronic lung disease

9. Dementia patients with acute changes in the clinical picture: Functional Assessment Staging of Alzheimer's disease (FAST) [19, 20]

2.6 Target groups in palliative care

The World Health Organization (WHO) Worldwide *Palliative Care* Alliance (WPCA) states the medical conditions that require palliative care as follows:

Diseases requiring palliative care in adults: cancers, Alzheimer's, dementia, cardiovascular diseases, cirrhosis, chronic obstructive pulmonary disease, diabetes, acquired immune deficiency syndrome (AIDS), renal failure, multiple sclerosis, Parkinson's disease, and rheumatoid [19, 22].

Diseases requiring palliative care in children: cancers, neonatal diseases, congenital anomalies, cardiovascular diseases, blood and immune disorders, meningitis, cirrhosis, AIDS, kidney diseases, and neurological disorders.

Persons who will provide palliative care to children should receive specialized training, and palliative care should be family oriented. Parents' comments on palliative care, taking part in the care of the child and being in a decisive position on legal issues, may cause disagreement with the team. Therefore, cooperation with the family is required. Families generally prefer home care after the acute period. In developed countries, this system is more suitable in terms of cost and compliance of the child. The palliative care team should cooperate with the family through home visits, educate the family on care, and provide psychosocial support to the family [8, 22].

3. Palliative care levels

3.1 Basic palliative care approach

It is a system where palliative care principles are applied by all health professionals and clinicians [4, 22]. Most patients with severe and progressive diseases are cared for by these clinicians in the hospital. Thus, this system focuses on the principle that all clinicians should have good knowledge and skills about the palliative care approach [23]. Therefore, these clinicians should be able to meet the healthcare needs of these patients who need palliative care [4, 22, 23].

3.2 General palliative care

At this level palliative care will be provided to the patients and their families by non-palliative care physicians and nurses who have palliative care experience. This understanding is defined as an intermediate level of palliative care, and a full-time palliative care is provided at this level [4]. These services can be provided in private centers or nursing homes. On certain days of the week and at certain times, a physician reviews the palliative care requirements at the care center where these patients are staying. He/she plans symptomatic therapy. Nurses work for limited hours in these centers. Other auxiliary health personnel also help with palliative care [23]. When complex cases occur at the level of general palliative care, these cases are referred to centers providing palliative care at a more advanced care level. This team also works as a local resource and training group [1, 17].

3.3 Specialist palliative care

This level of palliative care approach requires patient and family care and support depending on patient needs and available resources. There is a multidisciplinary approach to health care [1, 23]. This is the branch of specialization whose primary training and service area is palliative care. This branch deals with complex patients who require more time and need more care and require higher education and more staff and resources [4]. Palliative care specialists and other healthcare professionals trained in palliative care serve complex patients who need more care in hospitals or palliative care centers and hospices. In developed western countries, physicians who complete their education as an assistant in palliative care or palliative medicine departments in medical faculties are entitled to receive a palliative care certificate. Palliative care professionals are assigned to palliative care services of university hospitals or other hospitals or may work as a consultant in these services. Palliative care specialists may be consulted for patients in the ICU or other departments [23]. This team also works as a national resource and training group [1, 17].

4. Palliative care delivery models

Palliative care is delivered to the patients via four main models [1, 17].

4.1 Ambulatory palliative care clinics

This care for outpatient patients can be delivered in inpatient units, nursing homes, or other units, and patients can visit these places for 1 or several days a week for palliative care. These services include services such as medical support such as blood transfusion, pain treatment, symptomatic treatment, social services such as shower and bath, physiotherapy/vocational training, rehabilitation, massage, or psychosocial and spiritual support [4]. These centers offer low-cost care; hence, these centers have come to the forefront in recent years. In these clinics, services such as symptom control and nutritional support are provided, and patients and their families are supported psychosocially and morally. Families of patients are also trained in care [4, 15, 17].

4.2 Home-based palliative care

Healthcare professionals or nonprofessional caregivers provide care to the patient in their homes. In this way, hospital-level palliative care is provided at the patient's home. Home-based palliative care is based on traditional medical care and a supportive institutional model (hospital) [1, 13]. The patient can reach the palliative care support 24 hours a day, 7 days a week. In the home-based palliative care model, symptom control and terminal care services and basic needs of cancer patients are available through palliative care units at hospitals [17].

4.3 Inpatient palliative care units

These are the units in a hospital where the primarily responsible official is an internal medicine specialist or general surgeon and recommendations and support are frequently received from specialized palliative care staff [4]. In recent years, an increased number of hospital-based palliative care programs have been available to palliative care patients. General patient services in these clinics may not be appropriate for cancer patients with specific physical and psychosocial problems and who require a specialized approach. When a patient's care at home becomes harder in the advanced stage of the disease, palliative care centers accept the patient and support both the patient and his/her family in terms of pain relief, nutrition, psychological and social support, care, and training of the family [1, 4]. These units have improved care quality and reduced care costs for complex, high-risk patients who suffer from pain and other symptoms and whose basic needs are not met adequately [1, 17].

4.4 Inpatient consultation services

Providing services through consultancy is the most frequently used information method from past to present. Consulting services are an on-demand evaluation and management service [8, 10]. Clinical care may be requested by clinical physicians or other health professionals according to the care needs of inpatients. In palliative care, inpatient counseling services are provided by an interdisciplinary team. The team includes social workers, priests, psychologists, volunteers and therapists, and primarily doctors and nurses trained in palliative care services [4, 24]. This system provides uninterrupted service every day and every hour of the week. It is advantageous for it to be cost-effective because it contains fast, low-resource applications [4, 8, 24].

5. Palliative care practices in the world

Throughout the history of humanity, all societies have endeavored to provide adequate care, support, and respect to patients and the dead. In this historical process, as a result of the ever-increasing innovations in drug therapy since the 1950s and the better understanding of the dying patient's psychosocial and spiritual needs, the foundation of palliative care principles was laid [4]. Hospices were first established at the beginning of Christianity during the Roman Empire. In the fourth century AD, these places were transferred to religious institutions. Although this tradition was tried to be kept alive in the middle ages, many of the hospices were closed or converted into monasteries during the Reform period. This continued until the nineteenth century until Jeanne Garnier opened the first hospice center (Calvaire) in France in 1842, dedicated to terminal patients [11].

The first modern hospice named "Saint Christopher," founded by Dr. Cicely Saunders in London in 1967, laid the foundations for palliative care in the world and inspired other countries and people. With this hospice, protocols for palliative care of terminal patients were identified, and the number of palliative care providers increased rapidly in the United Kingdom and other European countries [25]. America and other western countries began to establish hospices for palliative care. Until the mid-1980s, the concept of palliative care was used instead of hospice care. In the early 1990s, the concept of palliative care was used for the care of individuals dying of cancer in America. Besides, individuals with other chronic diseases such as heart failure and lung disease also began to benefit from palliative care. Palliative care began to develop as a special branch in the mid-1990s and currently covers the care of patients with chronic diseases [4, 10, 26]. Over time, the understanding of palliative care has changed. Following this, the WHO defined palliative care and in 2004 published the "National Palliative Care Guidelines." Due to the need for palliative care and the need to provide effective care for patients, an independent area of expertise called "palliative medicine" was introduced in the United Kingdom, and specialists were trained in this field [25].

The European Association for Palliative Care demands formal certification programs and expertise in palliative care from policymakers and national councils. The European Association for Palliative Care conducts studies on training in palliative care and publishes guidelines on this issue. Through palliative care training manual for nurses [17, 25] and a guide to developing palliative care training in medical education, issues to be considered in palliative care training (palliative care and its importance; management of pain and other symptoms; psychosocial and spiritual care; ethical and legal issues in palliative care; communication and teamwork) by universities were identified [17, 27, 28].

The first palliative care in Germany began in 1983 with the establishment of a palliative service in the surgical department of the University of Cologne. The number of palliative care centers increased rapidly with the launch of a sample study by the German Ministry of Health between 1991 and 1996. According to Germany's 2005 data on palliative care, 111 hospice services, 131 hospices with beds, palliative care units in 116 hospitals, and 40 home-based palliative care services are actively performed [17, 29].

Italy is the leading country in palliative care, professional training, and research. The Academy of Palliative Medical Sciences in Bologna has been carrying out the necessary educational activities for the development of PC culture since 2007. The academy strengthened many international cooperation programs to be active in PC training activities [8, 10, 19]. To develop specialist nurses who have palliative care qualities and can provide the best palliative care services with evidence-based practices, Australia established a palliative care curriculum for nursing education and integrated palliative care into the undergraduate curriculum [10, 17].

Palliative care covers many disciplines. The palliative care process, which is developed parallel to the prevalence of cancer in the world, is carried out in different levels in developed and developing countries. Some countries where palliative care is considered a separate area of expertise include the United States, the United Kingdom, Canada, and Australia. There are guidelines for the treatment of different symptoms (bone pain, neuropathic pain, vomiting, depression, dyspnea, muscle spasm, terminal delirium, etc.). The American Medical Association applies a training program for end-of-life care for doctors and nurses. These programs include standards for the control of symptoms (pain, delirium, dyspnea anxiety, etc.) seen in the terminal stage [17, 27, 29].

The American Medical Association applies a training program for end-of-life care for doctors and nurses. These programs include standards for the control of symptoms seen in the terminal stage. Harvard University's Palliative Care Center organizes regular programs for nurses and doctors on palliative care. These programs aim to create awareness of interdisciplinary palliative care and to train educators specializing in palliative care [4, 10, 17]. Harvard University's Palliative Care Center organizes regular programs for nurses and physicians on palliative care to create an interdisciplinary palliative care awareness and train trainers who are specialized in palliative care [4, 17, 27]. Harvard University created the "Palliative and End-of-Life Care Training Project" in 1997 to train health professionals and increase their clinical competence in palliative care. This project was supported by the American Medical Association, the Robert Wood Johnson Foundation, the National Cancer Institute of America, and some national organizations, and more than 2000 trainers in 16 countries have received training under this project to this day. With a distance education program of 16 modules, the training program for health professionals has been continuing for about 17 years [10, 17, 30].

The Middle East Cancer Consortium organizes postgraduate courses for health professionals from member countries such as Cyprus, Israel, and Jordan. In undergraduate nursing education in Israel and Jordan, palliative care is part of clinical education. In the Arodaphnousa Hospice in Nicosia in Cyprus, the second and third year nursing students practice for 2 weeks. There are plans to make palliative care a minor in Israel [4, 17, 28].

5.1 Palliative care criteria of the worldwide palliative care alliance

According to the Worldwide Palliative Care Alliance (WPCA) 2014 report, 234 countries in the world have been classified in 4 groups that have sub-groups according to palliative care development. The WPCA has classified palliative care according to the following criteria [8, 22]:

- Palliative care throughout the country
- Comprehensive palliative care service integrated into the health system
- The inclusion of palliative care in general public health policies and transferring funds from other funds
- Participation of health personnel and local associations
- Effective and continuous palliative care policies
- Advanced and defined palliative care training systems
- Availability of morphine
- Palliative care awareness in the local community and health personnel
- Academic cooperation with universities
- National palliative care associations

5.2 Palliative care service classification

Today, palliative care services vary according to the level of development of countries as seen below [4, 8, 17, 28].

Group 1 countries whose hospice-palliative care activities are unknown: this group includes 75 countries (32%) such as Afghanistan, Chad, Guinea, Comoros, Korea, Libya, and Uzbekistan. There is no hospice-palliative care in these countries. Also, these countries do not have any palliative care policies that cover the whole country [4, 8, 17, 28].

Group 2 countries whose hospice-palliative care services are being developed: this group includes 23 countries (10%) such as Azerbaijan, Bolivia, Algeria, Haiti,

Montenegro, and the Vatican. There are no active palliative care units in these countries. However, efforts are being to establish palliative care services [4, 8, 17, 28].

Group 3 countries which have only local palliative care services and hospices:

Group 3A countries: these countries have an insufficient number of localized clinics and low-capacity palliative care. These units are not integrated into the health system and are mostly funded by personal donations. Morphine availability is limited. Governments do not adequately support palliative care activities. This group includes 74 countries (31.6%), including Angola, Bahrain, Bangladesh, Brazil, Bulgaria, Iran, Kuwait, Lebanon, Mozambique, Paraguay, and Sudan [4, 8, 17, 28].

Group 3B countries: localized palliative care services are not integrated with the general health system. Financial resources are personal donations, public and private health insurance, and local government resources. There are limited educational activities carried out by associations. Morphine is easily accessible. This group includes 17 countries (7.3%). Some of them are Portugal, Cyprus, Argentina, Malta Turkey, India, Nepal, Lithuania, Croatia Bosnia, and Herzegovina [4, 8, 17, 28].

Group 4 countries with hospice-palliative care services integrated into a health system:

Group 4A countries: several palliative care services are shared in these countries. Healthcare staff and people are aware of the importance of palliative care in these countries. Morphine and strong analgesics are easily accessible. These countries have limited palliative care policies and national palliative care associations. This group includes 25 countries (10.7%). Some of these are Costa Rica, Kenya, China, Denmark, Israel, Finland, Hungary, New Zealand, Malaysia, Mongolia, the Netherlands, and Spain [4, 8, 17, 28].

Group 4B countries: this group includes 20 countries (8.6%). Comprehensive palliative care services are available throughout these countries. These countries have active palliative care policies. There are advanced palliative care education systems and national palliative care associations that cooperate with universities. Some of these countries are Romania, Singapore, Sweden, Switzerland, Uganda, the United Kingdom, the United States, Australia, Iceland, Austria, Belgium, Canada, France, Germany, Hong Kong, Poland, Ireland, Italy, Japan, and Norway [4, 8, 17, 28].

In developed countries, a comprehensive palliative care service is available, while in developing countries, palliative care is under development. According to the WHO-WPCA 2014 report, in 2006, 21 countries (9%) had hospice-palliative care units, while in 2011, 136 (58%) of 234 countries had 1 or more palliative care units [8, 30]. The report indicates that there were positive developments in palliative care services in 2013. Seventy-five countries do not have palliative care; in 23 countries, palliative care services are being developed; 91 countries provide palliative care through local services; and 45 countries provide palliative care services integrated to health services. In short, developments are continuing in palliative care services in many countries of the world [17].

6. Palliative care practices in Turkey

The first step of palliative care in Turkey was performed by the Ministry of Health Department of Cancer Control in 2008: to eliminate the problems related to palliative care, the relevant units of the Ministry prepared a project called "Palli-Turk" with the contribution of many institutions, especially the WHO, and launched this project as of 2011 [11, 31, 32].

Nowadays, the increase in the number of palliative care centers is of great importance for the patients and their relatives. The Ministry of Health supports these centers both in terms of institutionalization and training of employees. For this reason, both the Ministry of Health and the palliative care association organize workshops and training programs [16, 31]. Moreover, guidelines prepared by the Ministry of Health according to the conditions and priorities of Turkey aim at identification and institutionalization of palliative care; development of awareness of palliative care, gradually increasing the number of palliative care services until 2023; creation of trained and experienced professional teams in the field of palliative care; and service to patients in need of palliative care. The reasons for the neglect of palliative care services in Turkey until today include family structure, problems in human power, lack of curriculum, lack of expertise in palliative care, and lack of awareness in health workers and patients [9, 33].

The number of palliative care centers in Turkey is not yet sufficient. However, serious efforts in the last 15 years have led to a significant increase in the number of palliative care centers. According to current data, as of May 2018, palliative care services are provided with 3971 beds in 307 health facilities in 80 cities [25, 33, 34]. The infrastructure and trained staff needs of these centers need to be prioritized.

Parallel to the developments in the world in the area of palliative care, the progress (although the level of education in developed countries has not been achieved yet) is continuing in the field of palliative care in Turkey. However, palliative care services in Turkey cannot be provided by expert teams. The teams that provide palliative care in hospital-based units do not consist of professionals who receive a training program at the level of palliative care expertise. Medical faculties do not include palliative care as a minor after graduation or as a graduate education program at nursing schools [4, 8, 10, 17, 19]. Curricula for primary medicine and nursing include only limited hours of palliative care training. However, palliative care services are in the process of development in our country, and health professionals (medical oncologists, nurses, and other health professionals) want to participate in postgraduate training programs related to palliative care [8, 10, 17, 35]. Also, palliative care training programs for nurses are organized with the cooperation of universities and hospitals. In this context, it is aimed to reach all nurses who provide palliative care services in 81 cities in Turkey through certificate programs.

7. Conclusion

In conclusion, a rapid increase in the number of people with chronic, life-threatening or incurable diseases, and health professionals' interest in the quality care of these patients has allowed rapid integration of palliative care, a new discipline, into other areas of medicine.

The main objective of palliative care, which is a philosophy of care, is to maintain the life quality of a patient in his/her last days when medical treatment is incapable and the healing process has stopped. Therefore, it is not the life span but the life quality of an individual that is important in palliative care. Therefore, the content of palliative care may vary depending on the individual's needs and the course of the disease. Today, there is a significant increase in the number of patients in need of palliative care, and this number is expected to increase further soon. For this reason, palliative care should be made in high quality and accessible all over the world. This can only be achieved through the development of national health policies, increasing the quality of training for health personnel, and further cooperation between countries. These steps will undoubtedly improve the life quality of patients and families who need palliative care.

Author details

Murat Can Mollaoğlu[1*], Döne Günay[2] and Mukadder Mollaoğlu[3]

1 Sivas Cumhuriyet University, Hospital of Medicine Faculty, Sivas, Turkey

2 Sivas Numune Hastanesi, Sivas, Turkey

3 Sivas Cumhuriyet University, Health Sciences Faculty, Sivas, Turkey

*Address all correspondence to: mukaddermollaoglu@hotmail.com

References

[1] WHO definition of palliative care. 2018. Available from: https://www.who.int/cancer/palliative/definition/en/ [Accessed: February 19, 2019]

[2] İnci F, Öz F. Palliative care and death anxiety. Current Approaches in Psychiatry. 2012;**4**(2):178-187

[3] Department of Cancer. 2016. Available from: https://hsgm.saglik.gov.tr/tr/kanser-anasayfadaire-faaliyetleri/palyatif-bakim/70-palyatif-bakim-nedir.html [Accessed: January 25, 2019]

[4] Tanrıverdi Ö, Kömürcü Ş. Structuring in palliative care units. 2016. Available from: www.solunum.org.tr/TusadData/Book/.../176201612846-_ [Accessed: February 2019]

[5] WHO palliative care definition 2018. Available from: https://www.who.int/news-room/fact-sheets/detail/palliative-care. [Accessed: January 22, 2019]

[6] Fadıloğlu Ç. Palliative care and evidence-based applications in patients with lung cancer. In: Can G, Aydıner A, editors. Palliative Care in Lung Cancer. İstanbul: Nobel Medical Bookstore Ltd. Sti; 2015. s. 1-20.18

[7] Boyle P, Levin B. World Cancer Report 2008. World Health Organization, International Agency for Research on Cancer; 2008

[8] Yılmaz A. In cancer patients receiving treatment in palliative care unit the Frequency of symptoms and palliative Care treatment in symptom control [thesis]. İzmir Katip Çelebi University Atatürk Training and Research Hospital Family Medicine; 2015

[9] Gültekin M, Özgül N, Olcayto E, Tuncer M. Current state of palliative care services in Turkey. Turkish Journal of Gynecologic Oncology. 2010;**1**:1-6

[10] Kıvanç MM. Palliative care services in Turkey. Journal of Health Science and Profession. 2017;**4**(2):132-135

[11] Bağ B. Hospice and preparation for death in hospice. 2012. Available from: http://www.akadgeriatri.org/managete/fu_folder/2012-03/html/2012-4-3-120-125.htm Erişim:19.02.2019

[12] Kabalak AA, Öztürk H, Çağil H. End-of-life care organization; palliative care. Journal of Intensive Care. 2013;**11**(2):56-70

[13] Aydoğan F, Uygun K. Palliative treatments in cancer patients. Journal of Clinical Development. 2011;**24**(3):4-9

[14] The National Consensus Project Clinical Practice Guidelines for Quality Palliative Care, 3rd edition (2013) Available from: https://www.nationalcoalitionhpc.org/ncp-guidelines-2013/ [Accessed: February 28, 2019]

[15] Clinical Practice Guidelines for Quality Palliative Care. 2018. Available from: https://www.nationalcoalitionhpc.org/wp-content/uploads/2018/10/NCHPC-NCPGuidelines_4thED_web_FINAL.pdf [Accessed: February 28, 2019]

[16] Demir M. Palliative care ethics. Journal of Intensive Care. 2016;7:62-66

[17] Şahan Uslu F, Terzioğlu F. Palliative care education and organization in the world and Turkey. Cumhurıyet Nursıng Journal. 2015;**4**(2):81-90

[18] Brinkman-Stoppelenburg A, Witkamp FE, van Zuylen L, van der Rijt CCD, van der Heide A. Palliative care team consultation and quality of death and dying in a university hospital: A secondary analysis of a prospective study. PLoS One. 2018;**13**(8):1-14

[19] Karadeniz Tekin N. Evaluation of symptom control in palliative care unit patients [thesis]. İzmir: T. C. Health Sciences University Tepecik Health Application and Research Center Family Medicine; 2018

[20] Şenel G. Palyatif Bakım Kavramı ve Palyatif Bakıma Kabul Kriterleri. Turkiye Klinikleri Journal of Anesthesiology Reanimation Special Topics. 2017;**10**(1):1-6

[21] Palliative care report at home and hospital workshop 25.04.2013, İzmir. 2013. Available from: https://www.researchgate.net/publication/320035280_palyatif_bakim_calistayi_evde_ve_hastanede [Accessed: March 8, 2019]

[22] WHO-WPCA. 2014. (The World Health Organization-Worldwide Palliative Care Alliance). Global Atlas of Palliative Care at the End of Life. World Health Organization 2014

[23] Gökçınar D, Kahveci K. Palliative care in turkey and world. In: Gökçınar D, Kahveci K, editors. Palliative Care. İstanbul: Nobel Medical Bookstore Limited. Sti; 2014. s. 2-3

[24] Wiencek C, Coyne P. Palliative care delivery models. Seminars in Oncology Nursing. 2014;**30**(4):227-233

[25] Temelli G. Perceptions of palliative care nurses related to death and palliative care practices [thesis]. Abant Izzet Baysal University, Institute of Health Science. 2018

[26] Elçigil A. Palliative care nursing. Gulhane Medical Journal. 2012;**54**: 329-334

[27] The European Association for Palliative Care. A guide for the development of palliative nurse education in Europe. 2004. Available from: https://www.eapcnet.eu/publications/Education/Nursingtaskforce/Recommendations [Accessed: November 13, 2018]

[28] The European Association for Palliative Care. Recommendations of the European Association for Palliative Care (EAPC) for the development of undergraduate curricula in palliative medicine at European Medical Schools. 2013. Available from: https://www.eapcnet.eu/ [Accessed: January 8, 2019]

[29] Bağ B. Palliative care practices in Germany's health system. Turkish Journal of Oncology. 2012;**27**(3):142-149

[30] Education in palliative and end-of-life care. 2014. Available from: http://epec.net/# [Accessed: December 14, 2018]

[31] TR Ministry of Health General Directorate of Health Services. Directive on the principles and procedures for the application of palliative care services. 2015. Available from: https://dosyamerkez.saglik.gov.tr/Eklenti/2817,palyatif-bakim-hizmetleri-yonergesipdf.pdf? [Accessed: February 19, 2019]

[32] Benli AR, Erbesler ZA. Differences on comprehension and practice in palliative care in Turkey. Türk Aile Hek Derg. 2016;**20**(1):5-6

[33] Turkey Palliative Care. Current developments, requirements. 2014. Available from: Http://Www.Arss.Org/Upload/Pdf/Dergi/2014_3edıtorden(121-123).Pdf [Accessed: February 9, 2019]

[34] TR Ministry of Health General Directorate of Public Hospitals Palliative Care Services. 2018. Available from: https://khgmozellikli.saglik.gov.tr/svg/palyatif.php. [Accessed: February 9, 2019]

[35] Özçelik H, Fadıloğlu Ç, Karabulut B, et al. Case management-based multidisciplinary care protocol in palliative care of cancer patient. Pain. 2014;**26**(2):47-56 Available from: http://Dergipark.Gov.Tr/Download/Article-File/95198 [Accessed: March 1, 2019]

Section 2

Palliative Care in Some Chronic Diseases

Chapter 9

Diabetes and Palliative Care: A Framework to Help Clinicians Proactively Plan for Personalized care

Trisha Dunning and Peter Martin

Abstract

The aim of the chapter is to provide a brief overview of diabetes and the associated morbidities that affect life expectancy to highlight why proactively planning for palliative and end-of-life care is essential to quality personalized diabetes care. Life expectancy may not be significantly reduced if blood glucose, lipids and blood pressure are well controlled; but several diabetes-related complications and long duration of diabetes affect life expectancy. Significantly, complications and related organ and tissue damage can be present 10–15 years before type 2 diabetes is diagnosed. The challenge of prognostication is discussed as recommendations for when to consider changing the focus of care from preventing diabetes complications to palliation and comfort care. Life-limiting illness and palliative and end-of-life care are defined. A framework for integrating diabetes and palliative care is proposed. The framework could help clinicians and people with diabetes prevent/manage complications and plan care to maintain quality of life, dignity and autonomy and ameliorate suffering as their life trajectory changes. The framework aims to facilitate care transitions and help clinicians proactively initiate management and have timely meaningful conversations about palliative and end-of-life care with older people with diabetes and their families.

Keywords: diabetes, complications, comorbidity, life-limiting illness, palliative, end of life, diabetes palliative care framework

1. Introduction

Diabetes is the most common chronic disease. People are at risk of diabetes due to genetic inheritance, epigenetic factors, age and lifestyle-related factors. The International Diabetes Federation (IDF) [1] estimated 123 million people aged 65–99 had diagnosed diabetes and predicted the number would increase to 438 million by 2045. Most older people have type 2 diabetes (T2DM), but people with type 1 diabetes (T1D) survive to older age. These data do not take account of the people with prediabetes who may already have one or more life-limiting diabetes complications at diagnosis.

An estimated ~ 20 million people globally need palliative care the year before they die; a further 20 million need end-of-life care per year [2]. The World Health Organization (WHO) estimated that 71% of deaths in 2016 were associated with diabetes complications. Most (~67%) occur in people aged 60 and older [3]. Therefore, older people with diabetes may have more than one life-limiting condition.

Aging is associated with reduced insulin production and insulin sensitivity that lead to insulin resistance, which increases by 1–2% per year [4]. Older age is generally defined as older than age 65 [5]. However, chronological age is not a good guide to disease, functional status, care needs or life expectancy. Biological age is a more accurate indicator of the rate at which body cells deteriorate but is more difficult to measure. Significantly, the individual's chronological and biological age may be different [5].

Many older people have several coexisting comorbidities/geriatric syndromes, including cardiovascular disease, renal disease, sensory impairments, lower limb pathology, cognitive changes/dementia, some forms of cancer and frailty that individually and collectively affect life expectancy [6–9]. Frailty predicts admission to a care home and mortality and increases the risk of death [10, 11]. Frailty is assessed in various ways, including phenotype and accumulation of deficits. The latter may be more useful to prognostication.

Many older people with diabetes have at least three coexisting comorbidities, but these are often managed as single entities that may not address the many diffuse symptoms [12–14] or the need to change the focus of care from achieving normoglycaemia to prevent complications to focus on comfort by managing existing complications and preventing hypoglycaemia and hyperglycaemia.

People with diabetes who can maintain near-normal glycaemia (~7%) and normal lipids and blood pressure are less likely to develop complications and may not have significantly reduced life expectancy. However, these parameters are often abnormal some 10–15 years before type 2 diabetes (T2DM) is diagnosed, and complications can be present and affect life expectancy from diagnosis [7, 12]. In addition, older people are less likely to benefit and more likely to be harmed by 'tight blood glucose control'. Therefore, blood glucose and HbA1c target ranges need to be individualized to minimize risk, especially hypoglycaemia risk and other risk factors being managed [15, 16].

Diabetes and the associated comorbidities affect the quality of life, compromise function and self-care and increase the need for hospital admissions and readmissions and eventually lead to death [11, 13, 17]. Over 50% of people aged 65–80 experience moderate to severe disability and increased dependency. On average, they need care 24 hours/day between 1.3 and 6.9 years [18].

Significantly, older people with diabetes and concomitant heart failure who have several recent hospital admissions and consult multiple prescribers are at risk of readmission within 30 days [19]. Hospital admissions near the end of life often result in burdensome and futile treatment that causes significant suffering and stress for the individual and their family [19, 20]. Likewise, people with cognitive impairment face many challenges, including decisions about their care.

Thus, starting conversations about the likely prognosis early in the disease trajectory can enhance people's capacity to make meaningful decisions and enable them to document their values and care preferences [21, 22]. In turn, clearly documented values and care preferences enhance family and health professionals' capacity to make care decisions consistent with the person's values and reduce decisional uncertainty.

2. Diabetes care

Quality diabetes care is described in many clinical guidelines such as the IDF [7], American Association of Diabetes/European Association for the Study of

Diabetes [23], Australian Diabetes Society [24] and Diabetes UK [25]. Many recommend 'relaxing' glycaemic targets in older people to reduce the risk of hypoglycaemia and its consequences: they usually do not include *comprehensive* guidance about other key aspects of palliative and end-of-life care. Exceptions are the IDF Global Guideline for Managing Older People with T2DM [7] and Guidelines for Managing Diabetes at the End of Life (currently under review) [8] and Diabetes UK [26].

Quality diabetes care encompasses achieving normoglycaemia (HbA1c <6.5 7%), controlling blood lipids and blood pressure using diet and exercise and commencing glucose-lowering (GLM), lipid-lowering and antihypertensive agents and other medicines when indicated, providing diabetes self-care education and undertaking regular health assessments. Self-care and adherence to recommendations are important to maintain health and meet metabolic targets.

Assessments could also encompass determining when the individual could benefit from palliative care and when to document an end-of-life care plan and an advance care directive (ACD). However, many clinicians find it difficult to discuss death and dying (giving bad news). Consequently, they miss opportunities to initiate conversations about these issues, and beneficial palliative care can be delayed [20, 21, 27]. Death cannot be cured: people's end-of-life can be made comfortable, dignified and consistent with their values and care preferences when these are known, clearly documented and communicated.

Many clinicians regard death and dying as treatment failure [28]. The terms 'failure' and 'bad news' are inherently negative. People often know they are not going to recover and want affirmation from their health professionals [28]. Some people express the wish to die while their identity and personhood can be maintained and not when they are terminally ill and incapable of making rational thoughts and informed decisions [29]. When such discussion does occur, health professionals often present the options as a choice between continuing and withdrawing treatment.

3. Palliative care

Palliative care originated in the 1960s and largely focused on end-of-life care at that time. More recently, there is increasing recognition that people with chronic disease could benefit from palliative care; thus the term broadened in meaning and scope to include non-communicable chronic diseases [30]. Most adults with chronic disease need palliative care as a result of cardiovascular disease [9, 11]. Diabetes is the leading cause of cardiovascular disease, and, in turn, cardiovascular disease is the leading underlying cause of diabetes-related deaths [3, 6, 31]. All health professionals who care for people with diabetes have a role in timely implementation of palliative care. Therefore, health services need to integrate such care into the services they offer and policies [32].

The patterns of dying are changing as more people follow the chronic disease trajectory, which is characterized by periods of deterioration followed by recovery until physiological reserves are depleted and the person reaches the terminal and end-of-life stages [32–34]. Many experts recommend palliative care should be implemented early in the disease trajectory, sometimes from diagnosis, for greatest benefit [30, 32]. In fact, Murray et al. recommend '[clinicians] should routinely and systematically consider whether our patients might benefit from early palliative care' [34]. **Table 1** explains the terms palliative care, life-limiting illness, end-of-life care and advance care planning.

Term	Explanation	Considerations
Life-limiting illness	The term life-limiting illness (LLI) describes people at high risk of dying in the subsequent 12 months. Many people admitted to hospitals and ICUs have a life-limiting illness. The Gold Standards Framework Proactive Indicator [33] outlines indicators of life-limiting illnesses for cancer, chronic obstructive pulmonary disease, heart failure, renal disease, neurological diseases, frailty, dementia and stroke Diabetes is not specifically mentioned in the GSF. It does mention organ failure, kidney disease, dementia and multimorbidity. Diabetes is the main underlying cause of renal disease, cardiovascular disease and some forms of cancer, frailty and dementia. Therefore, it is often unclear what 'initial' disease commenced the underlying pathological changes, which could be an inflammatory process related to obesity	Diabetes experts recommend normalizing blood glucose, lipids and blood pressure to reduce the risk of complications that can reduce life expectancy Palliative care experts and many geriatricians recommend people to document their values and end-of-life preferences while they are able to make informed, autonomous decisions Fewer than 50% of people with life-limiting illnesses actually have documented goals of care, and < 24% has documented care goals [36]
Palliative care	The aim of palliative care is to improve the quality of life, relieve suffering and manage distressing symptoms Palliative care involves symptom management, prognostication, advance care planning and transition to the dying/terminal stage [36] Palliative care can be used at any time and can complement usual diabetes care. Palliative care should be commenced early for maximum benefit to archive these aims [3, 31]. Early palliative care also increases satisfaction with care [34]	Many older people with diabetes could benefit from combining palliative care into their usual diabetes care as function changes and the burden of medicines and complications increase They also benefit from the support to document advance care directives much earlier than it currently occurs [36, 37] Good communication is essential to support older people to make informed decisions and to document their values and care preferences and goals
End-of-life care	The last 12 months of life and includes imminent death in a few hours or days [2, 30, 33] Four phases are described: stable, unstable, deteriorating, terminal [38]	Many people want to die at home, but most older people with multiple comorbidities die in hospital [39] Recognize/diagnose dying Identify whether unstable disease is likely to be remediable or likely to continue to deteriorate and progress to the terminal stage Treat or implement end-of-life care
Advance care directive (ACD)	Advance care planning (ACP) is the process used to develop and ACD ACD is a document that clearly describes an individual's values and the type of treatment they want if they are not capable of deciding for themselves and guides their medical treatment decision-maker and clinicians to make decision on their behalf that accord with their values and care preference [40] ACDs are often first documented when the individual has a rapid response team (RRT) call to assess sudden deterioration [41, 42] It is important to consider cultural and religious conventions when discussing ACDs. These differ among cultures and within cultures and influence laws and regulations and the way individual's view end of life and ACDs	Important information for older people with diabetes to document in their ACD are the things they value and give meaning and purpose to their life (values directive), the care they *want* to receive and the care they *do not want* to receive [40]. Generally the ACD does not have to be completed all at once. Older people need time to think about the issue and discuss them with relevant people. So, start the conversation and follow up at a later time It is important to check the persons' care preferences as part of ongoing care because they can change over time. Values remain relatively constant

Table 1.
Explanation of the terms life-limiting illness, palliative care, end-of-life care and advance care directives.

4. Diagnostic uncertainty and prognostic challenges: Challenges to discussing palliative and end-of-life care

It is certain that everybody will die eventually. The uncertainty lies in when and how an individual will die. The trajectory to death for people with diabetes can be a long and healthy one but is often a long process of physical and social decline followed by recovery until the final stages of life: the so-called chronic disease trajectory [2, 43, 44]. People can die, seemingly suddenly, during a disease exacerbation. However, most of these people have one or more indicators of limited life expectancy. Thus, their death was *possibly* predictable: the time of death might not have been. Episodes of deterioration become increasingly frequent over time and reduce the remaining physiological reserve and the person's ability to recover from subsequent exacerbations.

The chronic disease trajectory to end of life is unpredictable and includes many periods of deterioration and recovery before death occurs [38, 43, 44], which creates a degree of diagnostic uncertainty for many health professionals, people with diabetes and families. The uncertainty is compounded by challenges associated with prognostication and, sometimes, from misinterpreting individual's questions such as 'how long have I got Doc?' Mostly the individual wants an idea about how long they have left 'to put their house in order' and 'say my goodbyes'. Such questions could be a cue to health professionals to begin advance care planning to document the individual's values and care goals and preferences. Some strategies to enhance such conversations are shown in **Table 2**.

Diagnostic uncertainty encompasses cognitive, emotional and ethical reactions, which are affected by the need to discuss care options with the individual

• Use a value-based approach rather than focusing on medical decisions • Conversations can be planned or opportunistic • If planned ask the individual who they would like to be present during the conversation and have all relevant information and documents ready • Ensure the environment is confidential and welcoming • Ensure the person brings any communication aids they need with them, e.g. spectacles and hearing aids • Present the information in easy-to-understand words and formats, and assess their understanding • Frame the conversation as part of the individual's life story. Use own knowledge of life expectancy in similar conditions • Recognize and respond to verbal, non-verbal and emotional cues appropriately
Some useful questions include the following: these questions should *not be used as a 'tick box' list*. They must be personalized to the individual and the situation. The questions need not be asked in any particular order • What do I need to know about you to help me give you the best possible care and advice? • What things make your life worth living or matter to you? Rather than asking about the quality of life. • What does suffering mean to you? • What does a good death mean to you?
Not interrupting the individual is a key skill
Older people need time to process the question in order to respond—a complex cognitive process, especially when the topic is emotive. Interrupting can cause confusion and change the discussion, and important issues might not be identified
Understand and accept that not everybody is capable of making informed decisions during a crisis and some people prefer certainty, i.e. to be 'told what to do'

Table 2.
Strategies to enhance conversations about palliative and end-of-life care among older people with diabetes, families and clinicians [40, 49, 64, 65].

and often their families as well as organizational culture and personal experience [31] and individual tolerance of uncertainty [45]. Some degree of uncertainty occurs in nearly every aspect of health care and influence clinician and patient outcomes. Types of uncertainty include disease, therapeutic (risk and benefit) and prognosis [46].

Informed shared decision-making requires the individual to understand their illness, their treatment options and prognosis. Clinicians may not be comfortable disclosing their uncertainty to the individual [22, 46] and may refer them for a second opinion, admit them to hospital and/or order a barrage of diagnostic investigations [47]. These actions may or may not be indicated/warranted.

Sudden, unexpected death occurs in ~ 25% of deaths [2, 20]; however, diabetes-related deaths are often multifactorial, which makes it more difficult to predict life expectancy. A number of changes and well-defined patterns accompany functional decline to the end of life. These patterns are described in a series of disease trajectories [43, 44]. Prognostic indicators, include the Gold Standards Framework Proactive Identification Guidance (PIG) [35], life expectancy and risk calculators, the Diabetes Complications Severity Index (DCSI) [47], Cardiovascular risk tools and life expectancy calculators. These tools and calculators can help health professionals tailor care with the individual and start conversations about advance care planning.

Some experts recommend using absolute risk to decide which people are most likely to benefit from treatment because it considers the whole person and their individual determinates of risk [48]. These tools do not predict death. They are a guide to self-care education and care planning.

General indicators described in the GSF that indicate palliative care could be beneficial include:

- Decline in health and function.
- Unplanned hospital admissions.
- Symptoms that are difficult to manage.
- The person becomes less responsive to treatment.
- Person chooses not to accept active treatment.
- > 10 Kg progressive weight loss in the preceding 6 months.
- Serum albumin <25 g/L—other guidance suggests <5% in people with sarcopenia.
- More than 50% have a significant life event such as a fall, admission to a care home or bereavement.

In addition, a range of diabetes-related factors associated with reduced life were identified in a targeted literature review [49–51] and include:

- Long duration of diabetes.
- Macro- and microvascular complications [49]. Diabetes significantly increases the risk of all-cause and cardiovascular mortality in men and women by two- to fourfold [50].

- Glucose variability (fluctuation between high and low blood glucose levels) and rapid reduction in HbA1c [52–54].

- Multimorbidity: 80% of people 80 years and older have an average of 3.6 morbidities [54, 55].

- Severe hypoglycaemia [56–58] especially in older people and those on sulphonylureas or insulin and those with hypoglycaemic unawareness, including dementia.

- Lower limb and foot disease [59, 60].

- Polypharmacy [61].

- Cancer contributes to increased mortality in T2DM.

- Comorbid depression [62]: it is important to recognize and explore suicide ideation; suicide is twice as common in older people, and depressive symptoms are present in 80% of people > aged 74 who commit suicide. The severity of depression is a determinant of suicidal ideation [63].

This information and other prognostic indicators can be used independently or together to *guide* discussions with people with diabetes about advance care planning, their ACD and when to initiate palliative care. Documenting and ACD are part of holistic, evidence-based quality care.

4.1 Strategies that clinicians use to reduce prognostic uncertainty

Uncertainty occurs in all areas of health care, not just palliative and end-of-life care. A number of strategies can help clinicians reduce decisional uncertainty. These include:

- Acknowledging their uncertainty to themselves, colleagues, the individual and their family [46]. Not acknowledging uncertainty leads to further uncertainty and other problems. Acknowledging it can help build rapport and trust with the individual and their family.

- Accepting that death is normal and being able to recognize common disease patterns and their consequences that compromise life expectancy, signs of deterioration and signs that death is approaching. Guidance concerning these issues is described in the GSF [33], Murtagh et al. [31] and a suite of three tailored versions of information for older people with diabetes, family carers and clinicians [64].

- Understanding that many people choose comfort and quality of life over a longer life.

- Being able to recognize deterioration beyond the clinical parameters used in acute care. For example, using the GSF, which recommends asking the 'surprise question': 'would I be surprised if this person died soon?' The answer, yes or no, can guide treatment decisions, including whether and when to implement palliative care and aspects of usual diabetes care such as HbA1c, blood glucose monitoring and other metabolic parameters and when to initiate conversations about advance care planning with the individual older person and relevant others.

- Developing communication skills and the confidence to discuss palliative and end-of-life care. These skills increase following communication skills training [65] and include asking 'good/appropriate' questions, listening to the answers and using relevant probing and clarifying questions when relevant; see **Table 2**.
- Understanding that ACP is an iterative process that can be achieved using structured ACP communication tools and processes.
- Consulting the individual's ACD. ACDs are an outcome of advance care planning; they inform clinicians and families about the individual's values and preferences and enable medical treatment decision-makers, family and clinicians to make decisions consistent with the person's values when they are unable to decide for themselves [40, 64, 65].
- Asking about subjective life expectancy such as will to live is a strong predictor of survival in all age groups and genders [66, 67].
- Asking questions about self-rated *future* health, e.g. in 5 years, and adjusting for known mortality risk factors [67].
- Considering the health and care burden of informal/family carers: their subjective care burden is linked to various health outcomes for the care recipient including mortality risk [67, 68].
- Considering relevant policies, regulations and legislation that apply where the clinician works [51, 66].

These strategies show that subjective information and shared decision-making is an important part of the health assessment and risk calculations. After all, death is a very personal experience. They can help clinicians can include palliative and end-of-life care in usual diabetes clinical practice guidelines, is important.

4.2 Some key diabetes palliative care issues

Figure 1 depicts a framework for integrating diabetes and palliative and end-of-life care based on function and the chronic disease trajectory. The information can be used as a basis for developing a personalized care plan and with usual diabetes and palliative care guidelines.

Commencing palliative care does not mean usual diabetes care is abandoned. All care must be based on the best evidence. Care must be personalized and, ideally, developed in consultation with the older individual and often their family carers. People with diabetes do receive 'usual' palliative care, but it may not encompass important diabetes-specific issues that need to be considered. Specific information about these issues can be found in Dunning et al. [8] and Diabetes UK [26].

4.3 Managing glycaemia

Preventing hyperglycaemia is important to prevent ketoacidosis and hyperosmolar states, both of which cause considerable discomfort and can be fatal. Likewise, preventing hypoglycaemia is imperative. It is often missed because of the changed

Framework for implementing diabetes palliative and end of life care to support function and personalised proactive care planning.

Diabetes trajectory	Management focus and care planning
Basically well and functionally independent Consider number of comorbidities Functional assessment, including diabetes-self care Hypoglycemia risk assessment Medicine-related adverse event risk	Usual diabetes management but consider whether HbA1c and blood glucose target ranges are safe. Preventative care: health screening e.g. for cancer, vaccinations and dental checks. Treat reversible inter-current illness including hospital admission if needed. Medicine review, diet review and tailor sick day and hypo care plans to individual risk Palliative care could be implemented with usual diabetes care e.g. to manage pain.
Declining function in one or more: Comorbidities Polypharmacy Foot leg ulcers Severe hypoglycaemia Depression, social isolation Frailty Falls Cognitive changes or dementia Social isolation Carer burden – a predictor of the care recipient admission to a care home Discuss stopping activities such as driving when applicable	Continue complication assessments and consider referring for palliative/geriatric assessment. Treat reversible inter-current illness including hospital admission if needed, (LMOT) but there may be some treatment limitations Assess frailty status before surgery and before and after hospitalisation Revise HbA1c and other target ranges to avoid hypo and hyperglycaemia. Consider discussing values and care goals and use them to inform the care plan. If the person elects to develop their ACD, regularly review it to make sure their preferences have not changed. ACD should be documented before admission to a care home. May need protein and other supplements if malnourished and losing weight.
Significant functional deficits Sarcopenia, frailty Falls Frequent admission to hospital or Emergency department Declining will to live Self-rated future health Carer not able to cope	Palliative care/geriatric assessment and review ACD Medicine review may continue insulin in T1DM, Consider stopping GLMs and commencing insulin in T2DM if indicated Check that ACD still reflects the individuals care goals. Offer dignity therapy if available

Terminal Stage

End of life and terminal care
Decide care according to the individual's values
Simplify medicine regimen and stop most medicines
Provide comfort care
Implement the individual's ACD
Pronounce death compassionately.
Support family carers – e.g. offer bereavement counselling

Figure 1.
Proposed framework for integrating diabetes care with palliative care that supports function and proactive care planning. Reproduced from Dunning et al. [72] with permission. The framework has not been formally evaluated at this stage.

symptomatology and can become chronic. Hypoglycaemia is a risk factor for frailty [69] and cardiovascular disease [70] and leads to short-term cognitive changes and dementia in the longer term.

T2DM is associated with brain aging and cognitive changes that affect memory and learning and contribute to depression in the longer term. Thus, blood glucose monitoring in a suitable regimen tailored to the medicine regimen and hypo-hyperglycaemia risk profile can provide important information about glucose variability, the medicine regimen and care needs.

4.4 Managing medicines: Pharmacovigilance

Pharmacovigilance is important and includes regular medicine reviews, stopping medicines and using non-medicine options where possible and selecting the lowest effective dose when medicines are indicated. Insulin might be a safer option than some other glucose-lowering medicines and can be used with a palliative intent, that is, to improve comfort by managing unpleasant symptoms associated with hyperglycaemia. Some medicines are diabetogenic, and it is important to diagnose hyperglycaemia caused by medicines such as glucocorticoids and manage it appropriately.

4.5 Nutrition and hydration

Undernutrition can contribute to frailty, hypoglycaemia, slow wound healing and falls and can be present in overweight individuals. Eating disorders, depression, difficulty swallowing and other causes can be present. Likewise cancer, thyroid disease and other diseases can cause weight changes. These factors highlight the value of comprehensive geriatric assessments and collaborative interdisciplinary care.

4.6 Family carers

Family carers play a vital role in the care of children and older people with diabetes by helping with diabetes self-care and other activities of daily living. They are at risk of sleep deprivation, reduced immunity, depression and unresolved bereavement after their relative dies [68]. It is important to monitor their health and provide counseling and support.

5. Summary

Long-standing diabetes and associated complications significantly increase the risk of disability and frailty and reduce life expectancy. Palliative care can be used with usual diabetes care. Proactively planning for diabetes palliative care is important. Diabetes reduces life expectancy and can cause significant suffering. Considering the indicators of reducing life expectancy and implementing palliative care early into the diabetes care plan has many benefits, including reducing the suffering and the burden on the individual and family carers. Atypical symptoms associated with older age can make it difficult to recognize deterioration and underlying causes.

People admitted to hospital near their end of life are more likely to receive burdensome treatment such as admission to intensive care, resuscitation, dialysis and blood transfusions that are often futile [45, 46] and distressing for the individual and their families. Health professionals have an important role in helping older people with diabetes to plan for predictable changes in health status and to initiate timely palliative and EOL care to prevent unnecessary admissions to hospital and/or invasive intensive care that have little benefit, even when it prolongs life, and may not accord with the individual's core values. It is difficult for health professionals and family to make care decisions when the individual's values and wishes are not known, documented and communicated.

Acknowledgements

The authors acknowledge the older people with diabetes and their families and health professionals who served on research advisory groups for their research. The Diabetes Australia Research Program funded the research that enabled them to develop a suite of information to help older people with diabetes, family members and clinicians initiate discussions about palliative and end-of-life care. It is referenced in the chapter.

Conflicts of interest

The authors have no conflicts of interest to declare.

Author contribution

The authors conceived and wrote the chapter.

Author details

Trisha Dunning[1*] and Peter Martin[2]

1 Chair in Nursing Centre for Quality and Patient Safety Research, Barwon Health Partnership, School of Nursing and Midwifery, Deakin University, Geelong, Australia

2 Regional Director of Palliative Care Barwon Health, Chair pEACH, Professor of Communication and End of Life Care, The Geelong Hospital, School of Medicine Deakin University, Australia

*Address all correspondence to: trisha.dunning@barwonhealth.org.au

References

[1] IDF Atlas 7th edition 2017. Available from: www.idf.org/idf-diabetes-atlas-eighth-edition

[2] World Health Organisation (WHO). Strengthening of palliative care as a component of integrated treatment throughout the life course sixty-seventh 2014 World Health Assembly April 2014

[3] WHO. The Top 10 Causes of Death www.who.int › News › Fact sheets › Detail. 2018

[4] Baruah M, Kalra S, Unnikrishnan A, et al. Management of hyperglycaemia in geriatric patients with diabetes mellitus: South Asian consensus guidelines. Indian Journal of Endocrinology and Metabolism. 2011;**15**(2):75

[5] Thomson H. How old are you really? New Scientist. 2017:28-31

[6] Australian Institute of Health and Welfare. Deaths among People with Diabetes in Australia 2009-2014. Canberra: AIHW; 2017. Cat. no. CVD 79

[7] Dunning T, Sinclair A, Colagiuri S. Global Guideline for Managing Older People with Type 2 Diabetes. International Diabetes' Federation (IDF); 2013. www.idf.org

[8] Dunning T, Savage S, Duggan N, Martin P. Guidelines for Managing Diabetes at the End of Life. 2010. Available from: http://clearinghouse.adma.org.au/home/guideline/index.php

[9] Jacobs E, Hoyer A, Brinks R, et al. Burden of mortality attributable to diagnosed diabetes; a nationwide analysis based on claims data from 65 million people in Germany. Diabetes Care. 2017;**40**:1703-1709. DOI: 10.2337/dc17-0954

[10] Theou O, Sluggett J, Bell S, et al. Frailty, hospitalisation, and mortality in residential aged care. The Journals of Gerontology and Medical Sciences. 2018;**73**(8):1090-1096

[11] Botes R, Vermeulen K, Correia J, et al. Relative contribution of various chronic disease and multi-morbidity to potential disability among Dutch elderly. BMC Health Services Research. 2018;**18**:24. DOI: 19.1186/212913-017-2820-0

[12] Kalra S, Sharma S. Diabetes in the elderly. Diabetes Therapy. 2018;**9**(2):493-500. DOI: 10.1007/s13300-018-0380-x

[13] Schiotz M, Host D, Christensen M, et al. Quality of care for people with multimorbidity. BMC Health Services Research. 2017;**17**:745. DOI: 10.1186/s12913-017-2742-z

[14] Brutsaert E. Diabetes Mellitus (DM) Merk Manual Professional Version. 2018. Available from: https://www.merckmanuals.com/...disorders/diabetes...disorders.../diabetes-mellitus-d

[15] American Diabetes Association. Management of Common Comorbidities of Diabetes. 2017. Available from: http://outpatient.aace.com/diabetes/management-of-common-comorbidities-of-diabetes

[16] Arnold S, Lipska K, Wang J, et al. Use of intensive glycaemic management in older adults with diabetes mellitus. Journal of the American Geriatrics Society. 2018;**66**:1194-1194

[17] Badger F, Thomas K, Clifford C. Raising standards for elderly people dying in care homes. European Journal of Palliative Care. 2007;**14**(6):238-241

[18] Department of Health. Victoria Improving Care for Older People. 2003

[19] https://www2.health.vic.gov.au/.../%7B8DF949D8-2851-4DFC-8B57-57A7E1C24E9

[20] Caughey G, Pratt N, Barratt J, et al. Understanding 30-day re-admission after hospitalisation of older patients for diabetes: Identifying those at greatest risk. Medical Journal of Australia. 2017;**206**(4):170-175

[21] Mannix K. With the End in Mind: Dying, Death and Wisdom in an Age of Denial. London: Williams Collins; 2017

[22] Dunning T, Martin P. Palliative and end of life care of people with diabetes: Issues, challenges and strategies. Diabetes Research and Clinical Practice. 2018;**143**:454-463

[23] Thomas J, Sanchez-Reilly S, Bernacki R, et al. Advance care planning in cognitively impaired older adults. Journal of the American Geriatrics Society. 2018;**66**(8):1469-1474

[24] American Diabetes Association (ADA). European Association for the study of diabetes (EASD) management of hyperglycaemia in type 2 diabetes: A consensus report. Diabetes Care. 2018. DOI: 10.2337/dci18-0033

[25] Standards of Medical Care in Diabetes—2018 Abridged for Primary Care clinical. Available from: diabetesjournals.org/content/36/1/14

[26] National Institute of Clinical Excellence (NICE) End of life for adults (QS13) 107. https://www.nice.org.uk/guidance.qs13/chapter/list-of-statements

[27] Diabetes UK End of Life Care Clinical Recommendations. 3rd ed. 2018 www.diabetes.org.uk

[28] Brown A, Sun C, Prescott L, et al. Missed opportunities: patterns of medical care and hospice utilization among ovarian cancer patients 2014. http://dx.doi.org/10.1016/jygno.2014.030090-8258@2014

[29] Pearson P. The Dying Often Know They're Going to Go. 2014. Available from: http://Stuff.co.nz

[30] www.stuff.co.nz/life-style/life/10539263/The-dying-often-know-they-re-going-to-go

[31] Balasubramiam M. Rational suicide in elderly adults: A clinician's perspective. Journal of the American Geriatrics Society. 2018;**66**:998-1001

[32] World Palliative Care Association (WPCA)/World Health Organisation (WHO). 2014. Available from: www.THEWPCA.org

[33] Murtagh F, Preston M, Higginson I. Patterns of dying: Care for non-malignant disease. Clinical Medicine. 2004;**4**(1):39-44

[34] Palliative Care Australia Standards for Providing Quality Palliative Care. 2017. Available from: www.pallcare.org.au

[35] Gold Standards Framework Proactive Identification Guidance (PIG) (GSF). 2016. Available from: www.goldstandardsframework.org.uk/PIG

[36] Murray S, Kendall M, Moine S, et al. Palliatives care from diagnosis. The British Medical Journal. 2017;**356**. https://doi.org/10.1136/bmj.j878

[37] Orford N, Milnes S, Lambert N, et al. Prevalence, goals of care and long-term outcomes of patients with life-limiting illness referred to a tertiary ICU. Critical Care and Resuscitation. 2016;**18**:181-188

[38] Mercadante S, Gregoretti C, Cortegiana A. Palliative care in intensive care units: Why, where, what, who, when, how. BMC Anaesthesiology. 2018;**18**:106. http://www.medscape.com/viewarticle/901421_print

[39] Zheng L, Finucane A, Oxenham D. How good is primary care at identifying patients who need palliative care? A mixed methods study. European Journal of Palliative Care. 2013;**20**(5):216-222

[40] Palliative Care Outcomes Collaborative (PCOC) PCOC Phase Assessment Toolkit. 2016. Available from: www.pcpc.org.au

[41] Sweriessen H, Duckett S. Dying Well: The Grattan Report. 2014. ISBN: 1-925015-81-4

[42] Victorian State Government. The Medical Treatment Planning and Decisions Act 2016. Melbourne: Victorian Government

[43] ANZICS-CORE MET Dose Investigators. Mortality and rapid response team patients in Australia: A multicentre study. Critical Care and Resuscitation. 2013;**15**:272-278

[44] Jaderling K, Bell M, Martling C-R, et al. Limitations of medical treatment among patients attended by the rapid response team. Acta Anaesthesiologica Scandinaviaca. 2017;**57**(10):1268-1274. DOI: 1110.111/ ass.12202

[45] Lynn J, Adamson D, Rand Corporation. Living Well at the End of Life Adapting Health Care to Serious Chronic Illness in Old Age. Santa Monica, CA: RAND; 2003

[46] Dunning T. The common disease trajectories: Are they relevant to guide care as older people with diabetes progress towards end of life care. SM Gerontology and Geriatric Research. 2018;**2**(1):1011

[47] Strout T, Hillen M, Gutheil C, et al. Tolerance of uncertainty: A systematic review of health and healthcare-related outcomes. Patient Education and Counselling. 2018;**101**:1518-1537. DOI: 10.1016/j.pec2018.03.020

[48] Han P, Klein W, Arora N. Varieties of uncertainty in health care: A conceptual taxonomy. Medical Decision Making. 2011;**31**:828-838

[49] Young B, Lin E, von Korff M, et al. Diabetes complications severity index and risk of mortality, hospitalisation and healthcare utilisation. The American Journal of Managed Care. 2008;**14**(1):15-24

[50] Nelson M, Grenfell R. Absolute Risk and the Individual with High Cholesterol and/or Blood Pressure 2014 Presented at the Australian Atherosclerosis Society and the High Blood Pressure Research Council of Australia, Sydney

[51] Dunning T, Martin P, Orford N, Orellela L et al. A Suite of Information: Palliative and End of Life Care: Information for Older People with Diabetes, Family Carers and Health Professionals. 2018. ISBN: 978-9923333-1-7

[52] Leon B, Maddox T. Diabets and cardiovascular disease: Epidemiological mechanisms, treatment recommendations and future research. World Journal of Diabetes. 2010;**6**(13):1246-1258

[53] Siegelaar S, Holleman F, Joost B, et al. Glucose variability: Does it matter? Endocrine Reviews. 2010;**31**(2):171-182

[54] Krinsley J. Glycaemic variability: A strong independent predictor of mortality in critically ill patients. Critical Care Medicine. 2008;**36**(11):3008-3013

[55] Huang E, Liu J, Moffet H, John P, Karter A. Glycemic control, complications, and death in older diabetic patients: The diabetes and aging study. Diabetes Care. 2011;**34**:1329-1336. DOI: 10.2337/dc10-2377

[56] Iglay K, Hannachi H, Howie P, et al. Prevalence and co prevalence

of comorbidities among patients with type 2 diabetes mellitus. Current Medical Research and Opinion. 2916;**32**(7):1234-1252. DOI: 10.1185/03007995.2016.1168291

[57] Singh I, Ahita S. Selecting best-suited 'patient-related outcomes' in older people admitted to an acute geriatric or emergency frailty unit and applying quality improvement research to improve patient care. Patient Related Outcome Measures. 2018;**9**:309-320

[58] Sicar M, Bhatia A, Munshi M. Review of hypoglycaemia in the older adult. Canadian Journal of Diabetes. DOI: 10.1015/1.icid.2016.10.004

[59] Cryer P. Hypoglycaemia During Therapy of Diabetes. NCBI Bookshelf 2015. Available from: http://www.ncbi.nim.nih.gov/books/NBK279100/

[60] Hsu P, Sung S, Cheng H. Association of clinical symptomatic hypoglycaemia with cardiovascular events and total mortality in type 2 diabetes mellitus. Diabetes Care. 2012;**36**(4):894-900. DOI: 2337/dc12-0916

[61] Iversen M, Tell G, Riise T, et al. History of foot ulcer increases mortality among individuals with diabetes. Diabetes Care;**32**(912):219302199

[62] Ndosi M, Wright-Hughes A, Browns S, et al. Prognosis of the infected diabetes foot ulcer: A 12 month prospective observational study. Diabetic Medicine. 2017;**35**(1):78-88. DOI: 10.1111/dme.13537

[63] Jyrkkä J, Enlund H, Korhonen M, Hartikainen S. Patterns of drug use and factors associated with polypharmacy and excessive polypharmacy in elderly persons: Results of the Kupio 75+ study: A cross-sectional analysis. Drugs and Aging. 2009;(266):493-503

[64] American Diabetes Association. Management of Common Comorbidities of Diabetes. 2018. Available from: http://outpatient.aace.com/...diabetes/management-of-common-comorbidities-of-diabetes

[65] Alexopoulos G. Depression in the elderly. The Lancet;**365**:1961-1969

[66] Busko M. Hypoglycaemia and 'Underutilized' Risk Factor for CVD, Death. Heartwire from Medscape. 2017. Available from: https://www.medscape.com/viewarticle/877259

[67] Coyle N, Nanna R, Shen M, et al. Discussing death, dying and end of life goals of care; A communication skills training module for oncology nurses. Clinical Journal of Oncology Nursing. 2015;**19**(6):667-792

[68] Karppinen H, Larkkonen N-L. Will-to-live and survival in a 10-year follow-up among older people. Age and Ageing. 2012;**41**(6)

[69] Zick C, Shaman K, Mayer R, et al. Family, frailty and fatal future. Own health and family health predictors of subjective life expectancy. Research on Aging. 2014;**36**(2):244-211

[70] Pendergrass A, Malnis C, Graf U, et al. Screening caregivers at risk: Extended validation of the short version of the burden scale for family caregivers (BSFC-s) with a valid classification system for caregivers caring for an older person at home. BMC Health Services Research. 2018;**18**:229. DOI: 10.1186/s12913-018-3047-4

[71] Abdelhafiz A, Rodrigeus-Manas L, Morley J, Sinclair A. Hypoglycaemia in older people—A less well recognised risk factor for frailty. Aging and Disease;**2016**(2):156-167

[72] Dunning T, Martin P, on behalf of the writing group. Guidelines for Deciding Palliative and End of Life Care with People with Diabetes. Rijeka: in Press; 2018

Chapter 10

Palliative Care in HIV/AIDS

Habtamu Abera Areri

Abstract

In the era of HIV, palliative care is important to improve the quality of life of people living with HIV. The core activities of palliative care are control of symptoms and psychological, social, and spiritual problems. As a matter of fact, people living with HIV have a high burden of physical, psychological, and social difficulties which require palliative care that is holistic care. This implies palliative care for people living with HIV improves their emotion, physical symptoms, and psychosocial and spiritual functions. It can be provided by trained healthcare professionals, families, and community caregivers. HIV care and treatment guidelines should address the principles of palliative care, and policy should be in place to enforce its implementation for improving the quality of life of people living with HIV.

Keywords: palliative care, HIV, people living with HIV

1. Introduction

Palliative care refers to the active total care of patients whose disease is not responsive to curative treatment to improve their quality of life. The main goal of palliative care is achieving the best possible quality of life. In the process of palliative care, the core activities are control of symptoms and psychological, social, and spiritual problems [1]. This implies palliative care is a comprehensive care to solve physical, emotional, and spiritual impact of HIV/AIDS has on a person, no matter the stage of the illness [2, 3].

HIV is becoming a chronic condition that needs prolonged medical individual-centred care [4]. People living with HIV have a high burden of physical, psychological, and social difficulties which require palliative care that is holistic care and is recognised by the World Health Organization (WHO) as an essential element of HIV care, from diagnosis to end of life. According to Huang [4], in the management programme of HIV, palliative care should be integral to alleviate the distress and helps the people living with HIV to lead better quality of life. This means, in the continuum of HIV/AIDS, people living with this condition suffer from symptoms that are caused by opportunistic infections, the virus itself, or the side effects of antiretroviral drugs. Thus, to improve the individuals' quality of life requires to focus on palliative care, and enforcement of its implementation is critically important [3].

More importantly, people living with HIV need palliative care for many reasons such as pain, cough, nausea, weakness, fever, diarrhoea, breathing problems, other comorbidities, aging, and complex decision-making. Palliative care for these populations is a means of managing these challenging experiences and minimising burden on hospital resources [5]. Therefore, in the era of HIV, compressive package of care is critically important and should be in place in all HIV treatment guidelines.

IntechOpen

2. Settings of palliative care

Palliative care includes a wide range of interventions to improve the quality of life of people living with HIV and their families. The delivery sites for providing palliative care include home, community, and facility based [6, 7]. However, it can be given based on patient preference.

Home-based palliative care: It is an affordable approach in resource-poor setting and plays a significant role for a large proportion of people living with HIV and their families. Most people living with HIV prefer home-based palliative care. It requires training and education for healthcare providers like nurses, medical doctors, and community care providers. The training should focus on:

- Clinical diagnosis and treatment
- Basic nursing care
- Procedure of referral for better facilities
- Communication skills

Community-based palliative care: These include clinics, day care centres, school-based clinics, health centres, and work place clinics.

Facility-based palliative care: These sites include hospitals which provide both outpatient and inpatient clinical care by trained healthcare providers in the form of follow-up and admission. The specific palliative care activities carried out in hospital (facility based) based are assessment, symptom management, and consultation; discharge planning for all palliative care patients; and education of healthcare providers throughout the hospital [6, 7].

3. Who provides palliative care?

Palliative care can be provided by several categories of trained healthcare workers like physicians, nurses, and palliative specialists and by trained family and community care providers. Each category of providers has a unique role and training needs [7]:

- **Medical providers:** The role of medical providers includes assessment, prevention, diagnosis, treatment, and management of pain and suffering experienced by PLWHA and their families. They can provide medical and psychological support including necessary drugs to control symptoms that occur because of HIV-related disease. Thus, palliative care should be an integral part of nursing and medical school courses. That helps medical providers to diagnose and treat people living with HIV and their families. For this purpose, training and education of medical providers is critical [7, 8].

- **Traditional healers:** These groups of healthcare providers are linked between medical providers and community care providers in many parts of the health system and critical in improving access to care. The traditional healers are familiar to the family and individual needs. It is simple for traditional healers to explain the meaning of illness and death for families. Therefore, it is vital to train and include traditional healers in palliative care [7].

- **Family and community caregivers:** Friends, relatives, and others in the community can be trained to ensure that the patient is comfortable. The use of trained community caregivers such as volunteers, medical assistants, counsellors, and family members could provide and create opportunity to expand the provision of palliative care in community setting. These trained community caregivers can provide basic care, support drug adherence, symptom management, referral, counselling on diet, and social support. Families and friends should be provided with support even after the death of the patient. Bereavement counselling is an opportunity to support the loss of the affected loved ones and to consider the future [7, 8].

- Palliative care should be included in the curriculum of medical, nursing, and other health professional students to ensure that healthcare workers are sufficiently prepared to care for PLWHA in all settings and are able to train family members and community volunteers [8].

4. Principles of palliative care

People living with HIV need palliative care for symptom management, psychological support, spiritual support, and end-of-life support [8, 9]. Therefore, to fulfil these requirements, the guiding principles are to:

- ***Provide relief from distressing symptoms to enhance quality of life***: There are many distressing symptoms occurring in people living with HIV which need serious effort to improve quality of life, regardless of the stage of illness.
- ***Integrate the psychological and spiritual aspects of patient care***: Since palliative care is a holistic approach, services should consider the physical, emotional, spiritual, and social aspects equally. Therefore, interdisciplinary approach of services should be provided to better address the diverse needs of people living with HIV.
- Offer support to help patients live as actively as possible.
- Offer support to help families cope during illness and bereavement.
- Draw on experience and communication between the patient and healthcare provider to provide the best combination of interventions and medications.
- Affirm life and regard dying as a normal process.
- Strive neither to hasten nor postpone death [2, 3].

The crucial elements of palliative care in people living with HIV are the relief of pain related to physical, social, psychological, and spiritual aspects and enabling and supporting caregivers to work. The ranges of palliative care needed for people living with HIV are:

- Pain relief
- Treatment of other symptoms like nausea, fatigue, and weakness
- Supports (psychosocial, spiritual, for families and careers)
- Infection control [8, 9]

5. Palliative care for people living with HIV

Palliative care is critically important for people living with HIV to address multiple problems related to the diseases, its medication, and complications like pain, drug adverse effects, emotional distress, and physical symptoms [5]. These groups of patients experience a high degree of emotional problems like anxiety, depression, and mental health problems compared to general population [10]. Moreover, it is important for people living with HIV because of the following dimensions [8, 9]:

- **Complex disease process:** People living with HIV are suffering from ranges of several complications and opportunistic infections and related treatment side effects.
- **Complex treatments:** People living with HIV need lifetime treatment for viral suppression and treatment for comorbidities which will also create stress on the daily life of the patient.
- **Stigmatisation and discrimination:** In many parts of the world, people living with HIV are still suffering from stigmatisation and discrimination.
- **Complex family issues:** The disease has a great impact on the productivity of the family. The financial burden will increase as parents got infected and progress to advance illness.
- **The burden on healthcare workers:** The healthcare workers face stress related to lack of resources, symptom management, and management of related complications.

6. Ranges of treatment needed for people living with HIV

Palliative care needs for people living with HIV are multifaceted, depending on many factors such as the stage of the disease, the health infrastructure or system of each country, and the socio-economic status of patients. People living with HIV need palliative care for symptom and other related problem managements. Globally about 5.7% of adults living with HIV are needing palliative care at the end of life. The government should integrate palliative care policy in the national health delivery to improve the HIV care delivery system [11]. The service delivery should be patient centred which should be individualised, flexible, and collaborative. Communication should be open that will facilitate for shared decision-making during treatment planning [12, 13]. Therefore, people living with HIV need palliative care for symptom management, psychological support, family support, spiritual support, etc.

7. Symptom management

The treatment of people living with HIV requires the balance between acute and control of symptoms. Many people living with the disease suffer from different symptoms including pain. The common symptoms that require treatment are pain, nausea, vomiting, diarrhoea, weight loss, sleep disturbance, depression, mouth sore, sadness, fever, cough, skin problem, and respiratory problems [14, 15].

The central focus of palliative care is symptom management. For symptom management, opioids are essential for pain management. It is vitally important to consider the WHO pain management ladder. However, the plan for pain management depends on the individual preference. Managing symptoms enables people living with HIV to function fully. The need for palliative care for people living with HIV arises from the disease and its associated complications like varieties of symptoms and side effects of the drug management [8].

Pain is the most common symptom patients are suffering from and for which they should be treated if they complain of it. It can be managed both medically and psychologically. Spiritual and emotional support and counselling should always include the medical management of pain of people living with HIV. Deep breathing techniques, relaxation, and distracting attention of patients will also help as relieving methods for pain symptoms [8, 16].

Nausea and vomiting are another common distressing symptom the patients need to get advice on foods and feeding habits. The patients need to drink water, tea, ginger, etc. to get rid of the symptoms. The person with these problems should identify and avoid aggravating factors.

Diarrhoea is also a common problem which needs management. It may be a side effect of antiretroviral regimens; other causes include Cytomegalovirus colitis, cryptosporidiosis, microsporidiosis, giardiasis, Kaposi sarcoma, and other infective agents. Oral rehydrating solutions should be given to prevent dehydration. Use oral rehydration solution if there is a large volume of diarrhoea. *Encourage the patient to drink plenty of fluids to replace lost water.* If it is not possible to get oral rehydrating solutions, local remedies could be considered. To prevent and control diarrhoeal symptoms, it is advisable to avoid eating raw foods. In general, for diarrhoeal disease management, it is recommended to increase frequency of food intake, such as rice soup, porridge, ORS, bananas, and other soups [16].

Mouth sore is perhaps more than any other symptoms that could affect communication as well as comfort of people living with HIV. A sore mouth is very common in palliative care and may be severe in people living with HIV. It causes painful swallowing which may be caused by Cytomegalovirus ulcers of the mouth or oesophagus, virus, or fungal infection. In most cases it can be prevented by keeping the mouth clean and moist and treating any infections promptly. Nystatin oral drops after food and at night hold dose in the mouth to allow it to act topically. For fluconazole 50 mg daily for 5 days, use higher doses (200 mg daily for 2 weeks) if patient has difficulty swallowing and you suspect oesophageal candidiasis. Rinsing the mouth with diluted salt water after eating and at bedtime is the recommended care for patients with mouth sore [16, 17].

Fever in people living with HIV infection usually suggests an infectious complication. It may be a side effect of antiretroviral regimens; if suspected, assess and treat cause with paracetamol or acetylsalicylic acid, and encourage the patient to drink water, diluted tea, or fruit juice frequently. Fever, cough, weight loss, and night sweats in an HIV-infected person may indicate a heightened suspicion of tuberculosis (TB). At all stages of HIV, TB must be diagnosed, treated, and controlled. If fever is persisting, palliative care team must agree to do all that could minimise suffering [16].

Weight loss is also another challenge in the management of HIV conditions despite the use of antiretroviral therapy. Resting energy expenditure is high, and, therefore, food intake should be increased to prevent detectable risk of death. There are different related factors with weight loss in people living with HIV. These include mouth sore, disease of the upper gastrointestinal tract, anorexia, side effects of drugs, food insecurity, malabsorption due to diarrhoeal disease, and poorly controlled infections [16, 17].

Sleep disturbance like insomnias, which is a subjective complaint of inadequate nocturnal sleep, is manifested as difficulty of initiating or maintaining sleep, early-morning awakening, non-restful sleep, or a combination of all of these. In many cases insomnia is a symptom of another mental or physical disorder which includes pain, anxiety, depression, drug withdrawal, and side effects of certain ARV regimens, especially those with efavirenz [17]. A general care for sleep disturbance includes:

- Assessing and managing the cause
- Reducing the intake of stimulants and avoiding alcohol near bedtime
- Exercising regularly in the earlier part of the day
- Providing benzodiazepines

Respiratory symptoms are also common problems people living with HIV are suffering from. For instance, cough or difficulty breathing may be due to common opportunistic infections seen in people living with HIV. Difficulty in breathing is a frightening experience due to fear of death. Therefore, as a general care:

- *Position the patient to sitting to maximise ventilation.*
- *Ensure good ventilation by opening windows, using a fan.*
- *Adjust activity to help slow and deep breathing* [17].

8. Psychological support

People living with HIV face different aspects of psychological problems that require different forms of support [9, 14, 15]. These include:

- Counselling and testing
- Psychological and spiritual support
- Preparing for death

9. Psychosocial and spiritual support

People living with HIV need psychological and spiritual support critically important for coping with the overwhelming feelings and the threat of death. Psychological support helps people living with HIV to adapt to the disease and its complications. People living with HIV should disclose and involve in networking to get support from family, peers, and support groups. A multidisciplinary team is needed to address various concerns of people living with HIV. Psychosocial support for people living with HIV should also address finances, housing, and assistance with daily living. Spiritual support helps them to understand the meaning of life and improves belief and their faith. Spiritual support is also considered as resources for self-managing for these category populations [15, 16].

10. Support for the caregivers

Caregivers are frequently feeling anxious or have problems with sleeping, as the person they care for comes closer to the end of life. Mild psychological distress is usually relieved by emotional support from health workers by explaining the physical and psychological symptoms and challenging beliefs about death and dying. Through palliative care application, healthcare providers can reassure the caregivers and that you can give them more information and support [9, 14, 15].

11. Preparing for death

Preparing for death starts with effective communication with the family. Starting to talk on distressing concern helps both the families and the patients regard will, care of families, and related costs. Discussing sensitively about dying and grief reaction is an important aspect of care for people living with HIV and their caregivers [9, 15].

12. Benefits of palliative care

The benefits of palliative care are numerous which include the impact of palliative care on physical, emotional, social, and spiritual well-being. Managing symptoms affects overall functioning and plays a role in supporting ART adherence along with engagement and retention in HIV care. Palliative care as a complement to other care may contribute to a comprehensive HIV treatment. It is also a cost-effective approach that helps to reduce disease burden. Routine implementation of palliative care could contribute to manage complications and, thereby, enhance overall HIV care [18, 19]. It improves the outcome for patients with HIV and may complement antiretroviral treatment by increasing adherence through better management of side effects from the treatment, providing holistic and end-of-life care when necessary. Overall, palliative care will provide the following benefits:

- It improves quality of life of patient and families.
- It promotes better health outcomes, adherence, and retention and prolongs survival.
- It causes patients to spend more time at home and reduces the number of hospital inpatient days.
- It provides patient, family, and caretakers satisfaction.
- It reduces overall cost of disease [15].

13. Establishing palliative care programme

The World Health Organization recommends three important programmes for effective national palliative care programme such as policies, education, and availability of drugs. Government policies must be placed to support palliative care. For the healthcare providers and other concerned palliative care, education must be available. Finally, for the management of pain and other symptoms, appropriate medications must be available. These three programmes are essential for establishing palliative care programmes [9, 15].

14. Palliative care policies

The World Health Organization recommends that all countries should adopt a national palliative care policy, ensure the training and education of health professionals, ensure the availability of morphine in all healthcare settings, and ensure standards for pain relief and palliative care are progressively adopted at all levels of care [6, 7]. Therefore, palliative care programme should be an integral part of the national healthcare system [HIV care and treatment]. The presence of appropriate policy helps to solve existing obstacle, access drugs, and facilitate for resource and funding. Public health approach is a key approach of national plan that can be established through home care and community support [3, 9].

Policies can be generated from various levels of government and public and private institutions, such as medical and nursing schools, public and private healthcare facilities, and community-based organisations [6, 7]. Key actions for policy development include:

- Identifying the role of healthcare providers.
- Training and developing capacity of healthcare providers.
- Offering access to a wide range of medications for symptom and opportunistic infections.
- Establishing evidence-based programmes.
- Working with other stakeholders especially key governmental officials to promote policies and programmes to enhance access to pain and symptom control medications. Availability and prescribing opioids require strong policy support.

15. Palliative care training and education

Palliative care training and education should be an integral part of nursing and medical schools. Educated healthcare providers can provide better palliative care. There should be also continuous professional development on the area of palliative care for caregivers. Its effectiveness for people living with HIV depends on the providers' skills and is only as good as the skills of its providers. Therefore, palliative care training and education helps its implementation in an effective way [9, 14]. The training programme of palliative care should address three areas: [1] attitudes, beliefs, and values, [2] knowledge base, and [3] skills [15].

The best training includes hands-on clinical experience under the supervision of a skilled professional who serves as a mentor and guides colleagues in every aspect of palliative care ranging from symptom management, especially pain control, to the art of listening. Healthcare professionals should get interdisciplinary training which also provides them an opportunity for establishing a team that helps them understand and respect each other. Training and education will avoid misconception about palliative care especially regarding pain management [9].

16. Presence of drugs for palliative care

Drugs used for HIV pain and other symptom managements should be available and regulated by government policies. The drug list for palliative care in HIV is basic and short, and it can be found on any country's essential drug list. However, availability of these drugs for palliative care may be hindered by government policies regulating controlled substances such as opioids for distributing and dispensing the drugs. Palliative care professional should also advocate for legislative or regulatory changes at all level to make appropriate drugs because some of the drugs may not be legal in some countries, for instance, opioids. Procedural barriers may also need to be overcome for drugs to people living with HIV. However, drug availability is not only dependent on appropriate policy and efficient procedures, but also there should be policy for efficient way of utilisation, and the drugs should be available all the time to patients suffering from pain [9, 14].

Symptom control medications in palliative care that include essential medications for opportunistic infections in each health facility are as follows: [1] for pain management paracetamol, aspirin, ibuprofen, tramadol, morphine liquid, and dexamethasone and [2] for other symptom managements amitriptyline, diazepam, phenobarbitone, metoclopramide, chlorpromazine, ORS, co-trimoxazole, flucloxacillin, fluconazole, acyclovir, clotrimazole 1% cream, and nystatin suspension and pessaries [20].

17. Conclusion

Palliative care is critically important for people living with HIV to lead better quality of life. It helps them manage pain and other symptoms, the complex drug treatments, and psychosocial impacts and helps the patients self-manage. Therefore, care providers need to be educated on palliative care and have favouring attitude to implement it. HIV is becoming a long-term health effect with many concerns. Therefore, people living with this condition need compressive palliative care to address psychosocial and spiritual concerns and improve quality of life. The courses designed for healthcare providers should consist of palliative care related to HIV, and training should be given for families and friends of people living with HIV for better support. There should be in place policy to enforce the implementation of palliative care for people living with HIV.

Author details

Habtamu Abera Areri
School of Nursing and Midwifery, College of Health Sciences, Addis Ababa University, Ethiopia

*Address all correspondence to: habtamu.abera64@gmail.com

References

[1] WHO. Definition of palliative care. Available from: http://www.who.int/cancer/palliative/definition/en/ [Accessed: October 27, 2018]

[2] WHO. Palliative care. 2018. http://www.who.int/en/news-room/factsheets/detail/palliative-care [Accessed: October 27, 2018]

[3] Simms V, Higginson IJ, Harding R. Integration of palliative care throughout HIV disease. The Lancet Infectious Diseases. 2012;**12**:571-575

[4] Huang T-T. Challenges and responses in providing palliative care for people living with HIV/AIDS. International Journal of Palliative Nursing. 2013;**19**(5):220-225

[5] Merlin JS, Tucker RO, Saag MS, Selwyn PA. The role of palliative care in the current HIV treatment era in developed countries. Palliative Care in HIV. 2013;**21**(1):20-26

[6] The President's Emergency Plan for AIDS Relief Office of the U.S. Global AIDS Coordinator. HIV/AIDS Palliative Care Guidance#1 For the United States Government in–Country Staff and Implementing Partners. U.S. Department of State Office of the U.S. Global AIDS Coordinator. 2006

[7] Currow D. Palliative Care Service Provision in Australia: A Planning Guide. 2nd ed. Deakin West; 2005

[8] WHO. Palliative care. 2002. Available from: http://www.who.int/hiv/topics/palliative/PalliativeCare/en/on [Accessed: October 27, 2018]

[9] Schietinger H. Supportive and Palliative Care for People Living with HIV/AIDS. Common Health Spring; 2005

[10] Peltzer K, Phaswana-Mafuya N. The symptom experience of people living with HIV and AIDS in the eastern cape, South Africa. BMC Health Services Research. 2008;**8**:271

[11] Jackson K. Palliative Care is an Important Part of the Response to HIV and AIDS Care. USA. 2015. Available from: https://ehospice.com/usa_posts/palliative-care-is-an-important-part-of-the-response-to-hiv-and-aids/ [Accessed: January 27, 2019]

[12] Collins K, Harding R. Improving HIV management in sub-Saharan Africa: How much palliative care is needed? AIDS Care. 2007;**19**:1304-1306

[13] Epstein RM, Street Jr RL. The values and value of patient-centred care. Annals of Family Medicine. 2011;**9**:100-103

[14] UNAIDS Technical update. AIDS: Palliative care. Geneva; 2000

[15] Family Health International. Palliative care strategy for HIV and other diseases. 2009

[16] Spencer DC, Rossouw T, Krause R, et al. Palliative care guidelines for the management of HIV-infected people in South Africa. 2018. Available from: www.sahivsoc.org

[17] African Palliative Care Association. A Handbook of Palliative Care in Africa. 2010

[18] Farber EW, Marconi VC. Palliative HIV care: Opportunities for biomedical and behavioral change. Current HIV/AIDS Reports. 2014;**11**:404-412. DOI: 10.1007/s11904-014-0226-8

[19] Too W, Seymour J, Watson M, Harding R. Palliative care for people living with HIV/AIDS in Uganda: An investigation of patients & caregiver's outcome and professional perspectives. Palliative Medicine. 2010;**24**:S5, Abs. 539

[20] Republic of Kenya Ministry of Health. National Palliative Care Guidelines. Ministry of Health; 2013